ALSO BY ROBERT MARTENSEN

The Brain Takes Shape: An Early History

A Life Worth Living

A Life Worth Living

A Doctor's Reflections on Illness

in a High-Tech Era

Robert Martensen

Farrar, Straus and Giroux

New York

Farrar, Straus and Giroux
18 West 18th Street, New York 10011

Distributed in Canada by Douglas & McIntyre, Ltd.
Printed in the United States of America
First edition, 2008

Library of Congress Cataloging-in-Publication Data
Martensen, Robert L. (Robert Lawrence)
    A life worth living : a doctor's reflections on illness in a high-tech era / Robert
Martensen. — 1st ed.
        p.   cm.
    Includes bibliographical references and index.
    IBSN-13: 978-0-374-26666-0 (hardcover : alk. paper)
    ISBN-10: 0-374-26666-2 (hardcover : alk. paper)
    1. Chronic diseases.   2. Catastrophic illness.   3. Medicine—Philosophy.
4. Medical innovations.   I. Title.
    [DNLM: 1. Critical Illness—psychology.   2. Physicians—psychology.   3. Attitude
to Death.   4. Biomedical Technology—trends.   5. Caregivers—psychology.
6. Personal Narratives.   WX 218 M377L 2008]

RC108.M373 2008
616—dc22

                                                              2008026050

Designed by Michelle McMillian

www.fsgbooks.com

1   3   5   7   9   10   8   6   4   2

This is a work of nonfiction. The names and identifying characteristics of institutions and
of individuals other than public figures and the author's family members have been changed
or otherwise obscured. Dialogue is recounted from the author's memory.

Dr. Robert Martensen's views in this book are not necessarily those of the
National Institutes of Health or the U.S. government.

To my mother,
Bernice Sommer Martensen (b. 1919), and
my late father, Lorenz Thomas Martensen, Jr. (1918–2004)

Contents

Preface

This is a book for those of us who face difficult choices about how to live with serious chronic illnesses or conditions. To become seriously ill—whether it happens abruptly, as it may with sudden disruption of one's circulation or breathing, or at an indolent pace, as often occurs with cancer, Alzheimer's, or the complications of diabetes—is to enter an existential zone at once dark and confusing. As one recovers from the first shock of bad news, anxiety about the future may crimp, even paralyze, the imagination. One may turn to beloved others, who are often right there and eager to help, yet feel acutely alone. Specialists are consulted and Internet search engines activated as one experiences—urgently—a need to learn a new vocabulary of disease terms and treatment options. Hard questions arise, yet few unambiguous answers to them come forward. Treatment interventions are selected and may work for a time—often an extended period—only to have their effectiveness fade. A disease whose disruptions may have been ameliorated reasserts its power, sometimes precipitously. I have written this book as a navigational aid for those crossing these treacherous waters themselves or facing questions of how to manage the serious illness of a loved one.

As an emergency physician, I have helped care for thousands of very sick people. Many suffered from some acute problem that quickly abated, either on its own or because of timely interventions. For many others, however, an ambulance ride to the emergency room and subsequent hospitalization was not a singular event but a recurrent process. In these chapters, which follow the life cycle of issues and decisions relating to serious illness, from diagnosis to end of life, I relate my medical encounters with patients, friends, classmates, neighbors, and my relatives. Throughout this book I have gone to considerable lengths to conceal the identities of these individuals (other than my family members) and the institutions in which they were treated. Their experiences demonstrate both nightmarish and optimal treatment scenarios, as well as some daily realities and ethical dimensions of medical care.

The first two chapters, which are intended to complement one another, discuss the situations of Marguerite and Mike. Each one by nature was extroverted, a "doer" who believed in serving others. Marguerite and her husband found their vocation in international work for the poor; Mike developed his as an emergency physician. They both found that they had a dread disease when they were in their prime. As they pursued treatment, Marguerite followed one path and Mike another. Their stories deal with belief, both their own and that of the doctors who treated them.

Chapter 3 takes up residence in intensive care units (ICUs), a feature of the hospital landscape that has gone from being rare in the 1960s to ubiquitous today. Betsy, a widowed heiress in her early sixties, and Ellen, a scholar in her forties, seem to have little in common beyond the fact that both spend extended periods in an ICU. Yet what they do share—belief in the primacy of maintaining personal control—turns out to have quite different consequences.

However vital a person may have been in his or her twenties or sixties, eventually one or another bodily system threatens to fall apart. When that happens, one must quickly come to terms with specialist medicine and its cornucopia of treatment choices. Eliza, the focus of Chapter 4, does quite well into her eighties, which is not unusual these days. But then she starts having difficulty breathing due to a faulty heart valve. Should she have it replaced or just make some adaptations and live with it? The chapter discusses how to make treatment choices when no choice can return one to one's previous state of health.

To talk of seemingly endless treatment choices is, from another perspective, to talk of unrelenting treatments. While one might think that adult patients who pursue invasive treatments with little or no benefit "right up to the end" are misguided—and offer them that opinion—most physicians do not feel compelled to stop them, for such patients have exercised their autonomy. Britney, the central character of Chapter 5, was not an adult, however, but a seven-year-old child. How she and other children are being routinely treated reveals serious limitations in current ethical approaches, as well as some unexpected consequences for both the very young and the very old.

Physicians and biomedical scientists sometimes present their key assumptions and findings as if they are the only legitimate means of understanding not just disease, but the human condition. The situations of Ryan and Caleb, two New England teenagers I followed in episodes that occurred twenty years apart, provide the narrative of Chapter 6. Each suffered a serious neurological impairment, and their experiences call into question some contemporary biomedical definitions of personhood, as well as the assurances that lie behind them.

People with limited innate capacities or serious mental illness, as well as those with no insurance and little money, have never had an easy time of it. If their social context is supportive, however, they may do very well. When others or social policies turn against them, though, the consequences may be grave. Chapter 7 explores how and why some vulnerable people are able to make satisfactory lives even as an increasing number of others are made to suffer needlessly.

Most Americans die in hospitals these days, and often their dying does not go well. Compared to those in other countries, older Americans dying in hospitals experience an extended and agonizing process. Sadly, many also die alone or in the company of paid strangers—the hospital staff—and not with their families. But dying, like being born, can also go well. Chapter 8 follows the last days of my father, an engineer who died not long ago in his eighty-sixth year. He experienced a better death, and this chapter explores what that entails and how it can be accomplished.

Throughout this book I attempt to strike a balance between reflection and prescriptive advice. Its form is hybrid: part memoir, part philosophy, and part guide. In the middle of my medical career, I returned to graduate school to study the history of medicine and science. For several years afterward, I combined my desire to care for patients with teaching and writing about history, especially the history of mind-and-body relationships and of ethics. Because

I pursued these activities in medical schools, sometimes in leadership positions, I have been privy to aspects of their inner workings. In these pages, therefore, I have tried to write as both insider and outsider, as a member of university administrations who uses the lenses of history and philosophy to explore some troubling aspects of what has become a biomedical-industrial complex.

A Life Worth Living

1

Trials of the Body

In my experience, most people with something worrisome about their health seek out doctors because they want to know the truth, even when it hurts. Then they want the best available treatment. For decades, patients who follow recommended treatment regimes have been called "compliant" among doctors and nurses. The *Oxford English Dictionary* gives one definition of *comply* as "bending to the will of others." But when it comes to living with a life-threatening disease that admits of no cure but many treatment options, what role does "bending" play for both patients and doctors? What does compliance mean when all of us live within a biomedical-industrial complex that has its own values, assumptions, and interests to promote? Though any one of us within "the system" may strive to behave with candor and mindful compassion toward everyone, including ourselves, does "the system" encourage either?

This chapter tells the story of a woman who discovered when she was forty that she had advanced breast cancer. But the challenges she faced are similar to those contemplating aggressive treatments for other life-threatening diagnoses, such as advanced cardiovascular disease and degenerative conditions of the nervous system.

MARGUERITE AND THE PILGRIM HOSPITAL, BOSTON

In ERs, doctors and patients ordinarily meet as strangers. I was a little surprised, therefore, one Sunday morning in Boston in the mid-1990s, when I got a telephone call at home from a new neighbor asking if I would see her when I next worked in the ER at the Pilgrim, one of Harvard's principal teaching hospitals. I had met Marguerite and her husband, Eduardo, at a welcoming party another neighbor gave for them. It turned out she was the younger sister of a college classmate with whom I'd stayed in touch. Perhaps it was the connection through her older brother, my college friend Hugh, that prompted her to call me that Sunday. On the telephone she said she had been "putting something off" and wondered if I would "check her out." She and Eduardo had been traveling—around the world, in fact—with their six children, and then with their move from Guadalajara and all, she had just been "too busy." I suggested that perhaps she might be better served by seeing a regular doctor, one with whom she could have an ongoing relationship. I'd be happy to give her referrals to excellent physicians . . . No, she wanted to see me. It was "probably nothing," but she did not want to wait for an appointment with "a strange doctor." "That could take weeks." I was on duty starting at three that afternoon. I told Marguerite the ER would likely be busy, but she was more than welcome to come in and that I would be sure to see her if she did.

Like her brother, Hugh, Marguerite was tall, large-framed, and sturdy. He had been a standout hockey player at Harvard; Marguerite captained her field hockey team at Smith. Still a vigorous athlete at forty, she said she did not pay much attention to bruises or other "minor stuff." Then she laughed, remembering when, the year before, her ten-year-old son accidentally landed on her foot during a family basketball game and she waited two days before checking out her soreness and finding out a bone was broken. Other than having had a lot of kids, which she and Eduardo started to do in their early twenties, and a couple of broken bones from sports, she said she had never needed a doctor in her life. And she'd delivered her babies the "natural childbirth way." "It was pretty easy!" As she told me these details, I had a better sense of why she had waited to see someone about soreness in her left breast, which had been going on for about three months. I wish she had not waited.

A patch of skin about an inch and a half in diameter on the lower outer quadrant of Marguerite's left breast was red and bore little ridges. It felt warm to my touch. Because it was tender, I palpated very gently; nonetheless, it was easy to feel a hardened irregular mass about an inch in diameter below the redness. The mass seemed fixed to her chest wall. Her other breast seemed normal, and I could find nothing out of the ordinary on the rest of her exam, including her lymph nodes. I had seen and felt enough, though. Her breast's surface patch of roughened and tender redness, coupled with the firm mass below it and the fact that the soreness had been going on for at least three months, pointed strongly to one of the worst diagnoses one can have: inflammatory breast cancer.

I thought that I could be wrong—it could just be a breast infection, a mastitis with an abscess. But I didn't really believe that, even as I thought it; I just wanted the likely truth to be different. One might assume—at least nonmedical friends have told me they assume—that those of us who work in ERs over time must become "hardened" or "jaded" by what we do. But when it comes to realizing that the patient before you likely has some dreadful condition of which she is unaware, I have found that assumption to be a myth for me and for many of the veteran nurses, doctors, and technicians with whom I have worked. Our emotional range, if I may speak for them and me, has grown with our age and experience, not diminished. In the moments that lapse between suspecting something very bad and delivering the news, the cliché about feeling one's heart sink comes close to a visceral reality. And the sinking usually happens whether or not I know—or even like—the patient.

Marguerite sensed the change in me as it happened. "What do you see? You think it's bad, don't you?" she blurted out as I palpated her breast. I demurred and said I'd like to complete her exam and then talk about what might be going on. When I finished and she rearranged her gown, she wanted Eduardo, who had been waiting outside the cubicle, to come in. They had been together since she was sixteen: "We're a team in everything!"

I told them what I knew and feared. The fact that her left breast's reddened patch was warm and ridged—the cancer literature terms it *peau d'orange* for its resemblance to the peel of a navel orange—was a worrisome sign. The underlying mass was not especially large, which was good, but it was not small, and its hardness and fixedness made me concerned. Although all of it could just be an infection that would respond to antibiotics, I said it would be a mistake to treat it as such. We should arrange for her to see a breast cancer specialist as soon as possible; right now, in fact, if we could find one on a Sunday. I would make some calls. Marguerite and Eduardo sat on the exam table and held hands as I talked. Then they hugged and cried and I supplied Kleenex and said I was so sorry.

We spent a few more minutes together that day. I was able to locate an excellent specialist who would see Marguerite the next day, which she appreciated. She and Eduardo decided not to bring it up with their children, who ranged in age from eight to eighteen, until they knew more, which I thought was wise.

They both talked about God, about how much they believed in Him. I had assumed Marguerite was Catholic because I knew her brother was and that Eduardo was Mexican by birth. What I only learned on Sunday was that unlike her brother, who limited his regular church attendance to Christmas and Easter services, Marguerite and Eduardo's faith ordered their lives. They had taken their children around the world with them, for instance, because they decided as a family to devote a year to doing relief work for charities. Neither of them needed to earn a living—ample trust funds on both sides had taken care of that. They elected early on as a couple to devote their energies and resources to making a difference for the poor. For Marguerite this meant using her training in anthropology; for Eduardo, his own in civil engineering. They had first worked for CARE and Oxfam, and now they worked for Catholic charities. It had been a wonderful life for them and their children so far—"a grand adventure." Now they were back in New England, the home of her mother's people, to get some additional training in their respective areas and for their younger children's schooling. So far, God had been with them every step of the way. "On my shoulder—always," Marguerite said. She said it so lightly, so easily, and I was happy for her in this. Upon leaving, they said they wanted to stay in touch and would call me in a few days.

A week or so later Eduardo phoned with the news: biopsy had confirmed the existence of an inflammatory breast cancer. Due to scheduling issues, it turned out Marguerite would be working with a different cancer specialist from the one we originally called. This new faculty member had been recruited from the National Cancer Institute for her adeptness in devising sophisticated clinical protocols for treating breast cancer. Eduardo said Marguerite took to her "at once," and they were grateful to be in the hands of someone so brilliant and up-to-date. It had been "quite a week" for them all, he went on, as he and Marguerite had talked about her situation with each of their children individually and also as a family. "Tears and prayers in abundance."

Marguerite's situation had been discussed with the Pilgrim's Tumor Board, a multispecialty conclave composed of oncologists, cancer surgeons, and radiation oncologists that meets weekly to make treatment recommendations for new and ongoing patients. The Tumor Board recommended, and Marguerite and Eduardo readily accepted, an aggressive approach. Because inflammatory breast carcinoma tends to spread early and wide, she would have a modified radical mastectomy of her left breast and a simple mastectomy of her right—unless, of course, the surgeons found something worrisome in her right breast, in which case they might do a modified radical there, too. Then, after she had recovered from the surgery, they recommended radiation for her regional lymph nodes and at least three rounds of new chemotherapeutic agents. All this would take many months. Marguerite was going into the hospital tomorrow afternoon, and her surgery was scheduled for the next morning.

"How is she doing?" I asked Eduardo.

"Marguerite is amazing, just amazing!" he responded, getting choked up. "I don't know where she finds her strength." And the priests and sisters at their church and children's school had been "wonderful." Marguerite was with their children just then, but he wanted me to know how much she appreciated my examining her that Sunday. He also asked if I would stop by and see her in the hospital after the surgery. He said Marguerite's mother and sister were coming to stay with them and help out. Eduardo closed with, "We're going to lick this thing!"

As he talked, and especially after this closing declaration, I wanted to say and ask many things, but I did not. Early in my ER career I decided I would not press my medical opinions on people who did not request them. If Marguerite and Eduardo wanted to know what I thought, one or both would ask, either directly or in a way that suggested they wanted my input. But they had not; they were content with their choices. My job, if I had one, involved being supportive; at most, I could serve as their cicerone to the labyrinth of our complicated hospital, but even that would require a hint from them. To do otherwise, I told myself, to attempt to insert myself into their intimate life, would be disrespectful. The last thing they needed was for me or any outsider to sow doubt. After all, Marguerite had been my patient for only a moment, I was no cancer expert, and they were getting the best of care.

Even so, Eduardo's closing declaration—"We're going to lick

this thing!"—disquieted me. As soon as he said it, I wondered how their cancer team had presented Marguerite's disease and treatment options to her. Did they—and this was crucial—present their proposed regimen of surgery, radiation, and multiple rounds of chemotherapy, experimental in this case, as likely to be curative or even as giving her a reasonable chance at a cure? Or did they say, as I thought they should, that they would recommend everything they could think of to make her remaining life as symptom-free as possible but that nothing would be likely to cure her or significantly lengthen her survival? I could not tell from Eduardo's comment. He may, like so many in similar situations, have been giving voice to his and his mate's hopes. Her physicians may have spoken with them about her likely course and expected length of survival in detail, or in brief, or left the subject in the air. But if Eduardo's optimism sprang from what he and Marguerite had been told by her team, then I felt the team was doing her a disservice.

Advanced invasive breast cancer, like most other advanced invasive solid cancers, is a terminal diagnosis. One may live for several years with many terminal diseases, including some advanced cancers, and these may be years of satisfying quality, but the underlying diseases eventually exact mortal tolls. One does not "lick" or "win the battle against" such a diagnosis so much as cultivate resilience in its presence. Tragically, Marguerite's variety, an inflammatory glandular cancer, typically exacts its toll sooner rather than later.

This is an empirical truth. Should they not have told her that? Or, to put matters another way, should they have implied or even hinted otherwise? That I even raise the question may distress you. One may feel that doctors ought to nurture hopes of cure in patients, especially patients with advanced cancer, regardless of their likely outcome. What else can these patients cling to if not hope of a cure or years of symptom-free remission?

During the next few months, Marguerite fared well. The fact that she was comparatively young—forty—did not bode well for her long-term survival, as breast cancers in women under forty tend to be more aggressive than in those who are older, but her comparative youth and high level of fitness, spunk, and general health made her recovery go swimmingly. There were no significant problems from the excision of her left chest-wall muscles and the lymph nodes in her left armpit and over her collarbone, and only mild fatigue from the regional radiation. Indeed, the next time I really spent time with her and Eduardo was when we were swimming—Marguerite mostly floating on a raft—with their children over a perfect summer weekend at her family's place up on Squam Lake in New Hampshire. Her brother, Hugh, was there, with his wife and children, too, which afforded a nice reunion for him and me.

Following church and a lively Sunday lunch, Marguerite invited me to go on a walk with her. She wanted to show me something. After ambling along a woodland path for perhaps five minutes, we entered a circular clearing. Around its edge grew fourteen more or less evenly spaced old-growth white pines. As we slowly made our way around the circle in their dappled shade, Marguerite explained that they were her "Stations of the Cross." Her great-grandparents had first noticed the circular configuration of the giant trees and cleared the circle between them early in the twentieth century. She said she could find peace in many places and moments, but she found it most easily here. All winter long, as she experienced the surgery and rehabilitation and then radiation, she took comfort in her memories of this place and looked forward to returning. And now she had, and said she felt blessed. She also told me she did not fear death, that she knew God would keep her close in whatever state she was. She was about to start chemotherapy—an experimental protocol—and her doctors were optimistic for her. Before we walked back, she thanked me again for seeing her that Sunday and for "being there" for her and Eduardo. For a person as vivacious and engaged as she was in the life of the world, Marguerite then said something truly extraordinary. Looking at me with her widely spaced brown eyes, she said that if she ever became widowed from Eduardo, which she doubted, and their children were grown, she planned to enter a convent, a cloistered one whose members devoted themselves to contemplation and prayer.

Even though Marguerite's regional nodes had been excised and the area irradiated, the fact that two nodes above her collarbone contained malignancy was not a good sign. Their existence put her disease by definition into Stage IV, the typical designation of a solid cancer's most advanced stage. Five years after receiving a Stage IV diagnosis, only about 15 percent of women in this group remain alive, and the percentage goes down if they are younger. Of those alive at five years, very few make it to ten, and many of them are sick much of the time, either from the disease or a combination of the disease and its treatments. Even more dismal is the reality that it is not clear that aggressive chemical treatments in advanced breast cancer (as well as other solid cancers) make a difference in terms of additional length of life.

The traditional standard of "success" for a chemotherapy drug is if 20 percent or more of the participants experience tumor shrinkage as measured by CAT scans and MRIs. But the brutal truth is that tumor response of this kind bears little or no relation to overall survival, though combinations of chemotherapy agents may achieve additive effects in terms of percentages of tumor shrinkage. Side effects of some chemotherapy regimes include profound nausea, hair loss, and compromised immunity, among others, and may not be easy to endure. Current regimes that incorporate Herceptin or other monoclonal antibody agents or kinase inhibitors like Gleevac, which were not available in the mid-1990s, are proving more tolerable. What remains sobering, however, is that despite all the effort and hope that patients and their families and doctors and have put into breast cancer research and treatment in the past one hundred years, those like Marguerite who present with advanced metastatic cancer probably do not live much longer than their early-twentieth-century counterparts. It is harder to determine whether they live better. True, in the past two decades medicine has developed effective drugs for nausea and administration routes for pain medicine. Then again, some treatment regimes for advanced cancer have become so aggressive that they generate the side effects that call for these enhanced palliatives.

Heroism, like martyrdom, has its place, to be sure, and I would not gainsay anyone's choice to enter either precinct. But I think we in medicine should be forthright in telling our patients the degree and extent of side effects that will likely result from treatments we propose. The corollary is that if we are asking them to participate in a study that may advance medical knowledge in general but will likely not help them, and that may in fact place them in more peril than they would be otherwise, then we should let them know that directly, face-to-face. Instead, physicians often satisfy their sense of disclosure obligations by merely asking patients if they have read and understood voluminous consent forms.

Experimental treatment protocols have different purposes and potential benefits depending on their phase—I, II, or III for clinical drug trials. Phase I and II trials, for example, rarely provide a benefit, never a cancer "cure," and may cause harmful side effects. Before leaving that day, I asked Marguerite and Eduardo if they remembered which phase of experimental chemo trial she had signed up for, but they did not, though they said it must have been on the consent forms. They thought the trial's purpose was to test a new drug's efficacy, but they were not sure. Because they did not seem to pay much attention to the phases of her trial, I reversed my earlier decision to stay quiet unless invited to make a comment at that moment. I suggested they might want to check the phase, as it would help them know what to expect. At that point Marguerite indicated with a nod and look at Eduardo that she did not want to hear more. She said she knew she was in for a "rough time," but she was "totally confident" in her doctors and their approach.

After a drug has shown promise in the lab and in animal studies, it is ready to be tried out on humans in the three phases noted above. Although many participants believe each phase tests a proposed drug's ability to provide a positive benefit, this is not the case. Though Phase I studies are not concerned with efficacy—the degree to which the drug works—they may reveal some in the course of their trial. Their principal goal, however, is to determine a toxicity profile—what is called the "maximum tolerated dose" of the drug or drugs. In order to determine this, small groups are given escalating doses until the highest-dose group experiences worrisome or intolerable side effects. *Intolerable*, by the way, often means "life-threatening." Except for those unfortunate enough to be randomly chosen to be among the highest-dose group of the three, most participants in Phase I trials do not experience life-threatening side effects. Historically, however, only 2 to 3 percent of participants in Phase I trials experience *any* measurable benefit, and the risk of serious harm is about the same. In any case, participants only receive one dose or cycle of the investigational substance.

Phase II trials use doses determined in Phase I trials to look for evidence of a "response" to the drug, which usually means tumor shrinkage in at least 20 percent of the subjects as determined by CAT scans and MRIs. Phase II trials also collect toxicity data. Usually they involve a drug that has not previously been studied in individuals with the particular variety of cancer under investigation. If the drug does induce a response, the shrinkage is usually short-lived and does little to alter the person's overall survival. Most Phase II trials do not provide their drugs long-term. In the meantime, participants in Phase II cancer trials may experience significant side effects, as they are being given the highest dose that the Phase I trial indicated as tolerable. Phase II trials, like Phase I's, usually contain a small number of subjects.

Drugs that show promise in Phase II trials may then enter a Phase III trial, which compares the new drug, often in combination with other anticancer interventions, against more established drug and treatment combinations. Typically conducted in multiple centers coordinated by a central clearinghouse, Phase III trials enroll large numbers of subjects, each of whom is randomly selected to receive the new combination or existing standard therapy. Those who happen to receive the new intervention often benefit, as it is usually at least as good as the existing combination, and sometimes it is better. The side effects of those who receive the new treatment are usually similar to what they would experience if they received standard therapy. Participants may or may not receive long-term therapy of either type, depending on the study.

Should you happen to look at Internet websites on breast cancer treatments and drug trials, especially those sites provided by nonprofit organizations that receive funding from cancer treatment centers and pharmaceutical companies, you will have difficulty finding descriptions like the ones I outlined above for Phase I and II trials. Instead, you will likely see something like the following, which comes from the 2006 website of breastcancer.org, a "nonprofit organization for breast cancer education." Concerning the Phase I, II, and III sequence, for example, they begin their FAQ section as follows:

> *Before Phase III trials, the new treatment has already been tested successfully in many patients in Phase I and Phase II trials. Phase I trials establish how a drug should be administered, how often, and in what dosage. Phase II trials provide preliminary information on how well the drug works, and more information on its risks and benefits. A new treatment is not even considered for a large-scale Phase III trial unless it looks like an improvement in treatment and seems to be as safe as the standard treatment.*

It turned out that Marguerite participated in each kind of trial, albeit of different mixtures, going from Phase III to Phase I with three combinations of chemotherapy.

Since Marguerite underwent her therapy during the mid-1990s, the rate of introduction of new cancer drug trials has increased significantly. In order to get promising agents through the lengthy development process expeditiously, the FDA and major pharmaceutical firms have encouraged expanding enrollments in

Phase I and Phase II trials. Occasionally, they merge the phases into one combined trial. For agents engineered with toxicities that tend not to cause wholesale cellular destruction, such as monoclonal antibodies like Herceptin and kinase inhibitors like Gleevac, a combination of phases makes sense, for the drugs are comparatively safe. By expanding the numbers of human subjects and combining the phases, one can find out a candidate drug's net benefits much more quickly than with previous trial methodologies.

An important cautionary is that net benefit is calculated mostly by comparing the candidate drug to standard treatment in terms of tumor shrinkage, not necessarily subject survival, though both Herceptin and Gleevac have demonstrated significant survival benefit for patients whose tumors possess the relevant receptors. Measuring survival benefit takes several years, generally five, which is another reason to combine phases when a candidate treatment exhibits early promise. Many researchers now avidly seek biochemical markers that will allow them to predict how a promising agent will actually affect survival or long-term remission. If such markers are found, they can shorten the drug development period by years, with obvious benefits for patients.

Although I had hoped to, I did not see Marguerite or Eduardo for several months. When I called on the phone, they just chatted vaguely for a few moments before saying they were too busy just then to talk. Perhaps they felt I'd let them down; perhaps they anticipated I would try to second-guess their choices; perhaps they just wanted to be by themselves. In any case, when Eduardo and I ran into each other once early that winter, he just said it had been a "struggle," without elaborating or inviting me to see Marguerite or ask for details.

In February, when we happened on each other again at the

local deli, Eduardo said Marguerite was going to try a new intervention, bone marrow transplantation (BMT) and high-dose chemotherapy (HDT). The logic for this approach derives from its demonstrated success in people with leukemias, which are liquid tumors of blood cell types, and lymphomas, or tumors of the lymph system, especially of children. In women with advanced breast cancer, the purpose of a bone marrow transplant is to prepare them for undergoing high-dose chemotherapy, which generally consists of cellular poisons that kill all rapidly dividing cells, whether cancerous or not. The overall goal is for the poison to eliminate the cancer. Because high-dose chemo also efficiently kills bone marrow cells, however, the transplant of healthy marrow that has been previously withdrawn from the patient or provided by a compatible donor becomes necessary in order to replenish blood supply and immunity. Once the transplanted marrow regenerates the patient's blood volume and immunity, the theory runs, she would be free of her breast cancer.

Although the combination of BMT and HDT dates from the 1990s, its extreme aggressiveness harkens back to the mid-nineteenth century, when modern frameworks for understanding cancer first developed. The idea then, which continues to inform cancer therapy into the present, was that, since all life proceeded from single cells that multiplied locally, even the unruly cells of a cancerous tumor represented a local process. Hence, logically, a solid cancer like breast cancer could be cured if one could extirpate or destroy the tumor before it spread too far. Intrigued by this notion, which came out of German research labs, various surgeons, notably William Halsted at Johns Hopkins, reckoned that if they were sufficiently "radical" (his word) in their extirpation of the local site, they might "cure" (his word, too) breast cancer.

Committed to science, they measured their results carefully. But because they framed even advanced breast cancer as a local problem, what they measured was the rate of local tumor recurrence, not long-term survival. Surgeons performed tens of thousands of radical mastectomies, and in the United States Halsted's model became the standard of care for eighty years, not least because his disciples ended up chairing many prominent university departments of surgery and pathology as well as advising the early National Cancer Society. They did not take criticism lightly, for they believed that finally, their *scientific* surgery had something to offer women with a dreadful disease.

If one accepted their premise that cancer begins as an aberrant cell that spreads locally, then their logic of radical extirpation was impeccable. The problem, as credible skeptics started to notice in the 1920s, was that the premise was wrong. Indeed, as English surgeon Geoffrey Keynes began to demonstrate in that decade, many women with advanced breast cancer who underwent radical surgery died of the disease even as their bodies demonstrated "no local recurrence." His studies, and later those of others, revealed that advanced breast cancer is not just a local process, and extreme surgery based on that logic is no better than a combination of lumpectomy or simple mastectomy and local radiation. And the latter interventions are a lot easier to tolerate. But by then, "radical" approaches to breast cancer had taken on the status of dogma, especially in America. Into the 1960s, domestic skeptics, such as George Crile, Jr., at the Cleveland Clinic, however solid their analyses and prominent their positions, were treated as heretics by the surgical establishment. (Neither Keynes nor Crile, however, ever lacked for patients.)

Thanks to Crile and several activist women with breast cancer—notably Rose Kushner and Rosamond Campion—mastectomies and lumpectomies combined with local radiation started to gain mainstream surgical respect during the 1970s. The logic of maximum aggression did not disappear, however. Instead, it reappeared in support of aggressive chemotherapy with various cellular poisons administered in combinations of the kind Marguerite received. BMT combined with HDT is only the latest in a long line of approaches that derive from the "cut, blast, and kill" models that characterize much of America's tradition of aggressive treatments for advanced breast cancer. Again, their logic is impeccable, but it may rest on faulty premises. Alas, though oncologists have performed thousands of these BMT/HDTs during the past decade, so far no convincing evidence has emerged that those who survive the ordeal, which carries significant mortality risk in itself, live longer or better than their counterparts who choose standard therapy. Indeed, many cancer centers have declared the BMT/HDT approach a failure and have stopped providing it. As of early 2007, however, some Internet descriptions of BMT/HDT, like those of the phases of chemo trials I mentioned earlier, give little hint of the risks and prognoses. Nor do they mention that BMT/HDT, being a procedure and not a drug protocol or device, is only lightly regulated by the FDA.

When I last saw Marguerite as a patient, it was not by appointment. About a year and a half after she first called me, I just happened to be on duty at five o'clock one morning when Eduardo helped her into the Pilgrim's ER. "I wanted to bring her earlier," he said, "but Marguerite wanted to see if she could make it. She didn't want to wake up her doctors." They seemed both startled and reassured to see me. Marguerite was alert, but barely. Her pulse was rapid, her blood pressure on the low side, and blood oozed from her chest wall and her anus. She had finished her BMT/HDT eight weeks before. She wondered why she had bothered with it, Eduardo said, for she had just gone from sick to sicker, with only brief respites and much agony in between. "Even before we started the last chemo, before the bone marrow transplant–chemo thing," he said, "we knew the cancer had spread to her lungs and liver and brain. Now she knows she is at the end." Then, his voice trailing, he added, "I guess the doctors tried their best, though it's been so rough. Had we only known . . . Maybe they tried to tell us, but we didn't pay attention." They had come in because of the bleeding. They needed help to get it stopped. Then they wanted hospice.

As we started emergency treatments for her bleeding, I paged the medical resident from upstairs to come to the ER, see Marguerite, and admit her. At the Pilgrim, as in some other esteemed teaching hospitals, residents admit all the patients and, except in the ER, write all the orders for their treatment and diagnostic tests. This has been policy for years. The staff physicians, even the most senior faculty, do not have the authority, at least nominally, to admit patients or to write orders. This resident, with whom I had crossed swords on other occasions, did not want to admit Marguerite. She started to give her reasons in front of the three of us and the nurse, but I motioned for her to join me outside the cubicle.

An assertive junior resident even by the standards of an assertive resident class, she told me she would not admit the patient. "She's dying," she said. She had treated Marguerite on previous admissions. "We've tried *everything*, and it hasn't worked."

"And so you will send her home to bleed to death?" I asked rhetorically.

"She's gonna die anyway, no matter what," the resident fired back. "I'm not staying up for this. There's nothing to treat!"

"Admit her," I said quietly. "It's the least we can do."

"But—"

Fed up, I played a trump: "Or I will call the chief resident at home, or the chief of medicine if I have to." Marguerite was admitted, and her bleeding was stanched for the moment.

Residents working in advanced teaching and research hospitals, such as the Pilgrim, are sometimes drilled and drilled again by the faculty and each other to think of medicine as a supremely scientific activity. Critically ill and dying patients are approached as if their situations need to be *just so* in terms of medical interest to make them eligible for admission. If the patients—or rather, their diseases—are not, or if their condition has progressed beyond any hope of remission (like Marguerite's), then residents and faculty with this outlook often balk at caring for them. It is as though the hospital has become a theater in which a strange inversion of roles has taken place: doctors acting as though the patients are primarily there to perform for them, when for patients and their families, it is the other way around. Patients, especially patients who live with terminal diagnoses, come with the expectation that a hospital's physicians will serve them when their need is great, not shy away when their condition no longer measures up.

After seeing Marguerite and Eduardo off to her hospital room that morning, I felt ashamed. Can belief in medicine as a profession whose principal value lies in its commitment to instrumental rationality—its science—at times verge on the fanatical? I have seen it happen. Sometimes great things come from such an approach— the development of some successful chemotherapy treatments for Hodgkin's lymphoma and childhood leukemias come to mind. But many patients can and do die along the way as the experimental approaches undergo increasing refinement. Marguerite was in the latter group. She was dying, and anyone could see it. That she was dying in a particular way as the likely result of treatments that probably did not extend her life one whit reflects the reality that for those who present with advanced solid cancers, truly successful treatments—those that produce cures or long-term remissions without serious side effects—remain elusive. But *she*, the person, remains present, and doctors work with people. How have we let the assumptions of biomedicine turn into an emotional carapace for our patients and ourselves?

After attending to Marguerite that morning, I rested in preparation for my late-afternoon seminar with Harvard undergraduates on the history of medicine and society in medieval and early modern Europe. Most of the students were premeds, and we had been exploring the history of our early counterparts' assessments of their professional roles. Medicine gained its status as a learned profession in medieval universities established originally by the Catholic Church to train religious leaders and church lawyers, and I encouraged the students to look across the disciplines for common themes. As we pored over primary texts from centuries ago, we began musing on how some physicians and priests then interpreted their roles in caring for someone under grievous threat either from a disease or from a diseaselike affliction. For a priest, whether or not an affliction shortened a believer's earthly life was important, but the crucial task was to preserve the sufferer's opportunity for an eternal life, which was then, at least in Christian culture, more important.

Suppose you were an ambitious priest who decided to devote yourself to understanding the inner workings of heresy and its counterpart, sanctity. Confronted with a suspected heretic, desperate to root out heresy and, if possible, save the individual heretic's chance for eternal life, how far should you go to investigate and treat the heretic's affliction? Is there a way, I asked the students, in which they could see the Church's development of inquisitorial trials, which began in the thirteenth century as a process for determining the character and extent of a person's alleged sin (or sanctity), as similar to a physician's aggressive testing of a compliant patient with a life-threatening condition? Although it might seem far-fetched, could they see an inquisitor's prescription of a trial of torture as a sincere effort on the inquisitor's part to save a life by intervening in a disastrous course—the heretic's progression to eternal damnation? Could they imagine that the inquisitor did not intend cruelty by prescribing graduated administration of pain, but rather that he imagined the process as an extreme but therapeutic trial?

At this point a few students seemed impatient, as though I had gone off the deep end, but most seemed willing to let me go on. Did they find it significant, I continued, that the first Church council to establish inquisitorial procedures, Lateran IV, which met in 1215, chose not to allude to the priest-inquisitor's semijudicial role, but instead portrayed him in medical garb?

> *The priest shall be discerning and prudent, so that like a skilled doctor he may pour wine and oil over the wounds of the injured one. Let him carefully inquire about the circumstances of both the sinner and the sin so that he may prudently discern what sort of medical advice he ought to give and what remedy to apply, using various means to heal the sick person.*

In the High Middle Ages, I reminded them, Church sponsorship of the early universities in part reflected a growing preoccu-

pation in Christendom with what constituted truth. An inquisitorial trial, like a legal trial or a medical investigation, was seen
by them as a process for proving the truth. Etymologically, the
Latin for generating proof—*probare*—also means "to test." A trial
of the body, if successful, would produce a purgative function.
God, through the mediation of priestly inquisitors, "proves" the
sinner through the infliction of suffering. If successful, the proof
purges an individual of sins for his or her own good. Or it sup-
ports the person's reputation for sanctity. Thinking at that moment of Marguerite, I added that these early inquisitions tended
to be directed at women known in their communities for being
spiritually intense. Were they heretics or saints? was the common
question. One of the realities of medieval pursuits of the truth,
including those common in inquisitorial trials, was that despite
the appearance of parity, individuals or debating positions that
challenged orthodoxy almost always lost. Those who asked the
questions—and the dogma that stood behind them—held most of
the cards, and they kept them close to their chests.

Then I mentioned how early learned doctors tended to conduct themselves around the seriously afflicted. Compared to priestly
inquisitors, physicians observed boundaries, and their patients expected them to. Patients did not assume that their physicians
would prescribe aggressive treatments when the outcome looked
doubtful; indeed, I showed them copies of early cartoons in which
the families of the dying are shooing the doctors away. Dying often happened over days or weeks then—contagious disease being
the usual culprit—and patients and their families consulted physicians for estimates on how long the terminally ill person might
expect to remain lucid. To that end, and to ease discomfort, physicians in the early modern period commonly prescribed laudanum,

a derivative of opium, for pain, quinine for fever, and alcohol-based potions. Patients desired accurate prognoses in order to plan for their families, consult with their spiritual advisers on affairs of conscience, and say a proper goodbye to their families.

As we usually did toward the end of our seminars, I then invited the students to speculate on the past in the present. How, I asked, might we characterize medical and religious approaches to life and attempts to save it today? In experimental trials of dangerous treatments for serious illnesses, how far should doctors go to prove *their* truth when it involves the knowing infliction of suffering on their patients? What obligations do physicians, clinical trial sponsors, and hospitals owe the afflicted if and when trial participants fail to respond?

As we had not been studying modern human experimentation and aggressive treatment, my students were surprised to learn that American cancer treatments for the past hundred years have tended to be more aggressive than European strategies, though ours rarely result in better outcomes. Then I mentioned that unlike in Western Europe and Canada, where religious outlooks have not dominated the public imagination for close to two hundred years, American religiosity—always comparatively intense, as early observers like Alexis de Tocqueville noted—is undergoing a remarkable upswing. Are we Americans just more dogmatic in general? A student commented that Massachusetts and Harvard were established by religious zealots, which elicited a few smiles.

Finally, one asked, "So what does it mean to be *rational* about medical treatments? I mean for doctors *and* the patients." Images of Marguerite as I had seen her that morning came back to me as she said this, although I did not mention her situation to the students.

Marguerite died a few days later in the hospital—miserably, I'm afraid, but at least with her husband and older children at her side. I had hoped she might have spent her final weeks and days otherwise, knowing she was dying, to be sure, but at home in reasonable comfort and with her family, perhaps even able to make one final visit to their place on the lake. After all, she did not fear her earthly death. Why did her doctors treat her as though she did? Why did they not make a point of knowing what mattered to her and adjust their trials accordingly? What were they trying to prove?

Had Marguerite stated her existential priorities forcefully and early on, perhaps her cancer team and she would have arranged her final months differently. But people who by nature or habit embrace compliance, though fully able to give voice to their inner sense in private settings, as Marguerite did with me in the New Hampshire woods, may hesitate at being candid in the unfamiliar and alien context of a hospital conference room packed with white coats known and unknown. Wanting to avoid being considered heretical, they may find it too stressful to dissent from the unspoken orthodoxy, which is that a proper response requires enlistment and reenlistment in an indefinite series of "battles" with an evil foe.

Recent proposals by FDA officials, legislators such as Senator Sam Brownback, and some drug makers to provide experimental cancer drugs to *any* patient with the requisite diagnosis, enrolled in a trial or not, put the question squarely before patients. No longer will physicians and clinical trial centers serve as gatekeepers, as they have in the past. As with AIDS drugs in the late 1980s and early 1990s, urban and rural patients will have an increasing choice of experimental treatments, which is good. The cycle of knowledge concerning what works and what doesn't will speed up, which is also good. But so, too, will the incidence of undesirable side effects, for it takes more than a few patients for toxicity profiles to fully reveal themselves. Long-term efficacy, by which I mean enhanced survival compared to standard treatment, will, by definition, take years to demonstrate. In the meantime, how will promoters present their new wares? (One can expect television ads if patient access expands as envisioned by its adherents.) In the face of little or no evidence of enhanced survival, will they be candid about the risks and modest benefits that such therapies may bring? If they are, will patients be able to hear them? Or will they give way, as many doctors already do, to a psychosocial imperative to pursue whatever treatments are on offer?

As one anticipates these likely shifts in the moral and existential calculus of what is "enough," other questions arise. How will doctors and families regard the afflicted person who decides "enough is enough" even as their televisions glow with additional possibilities? Will we fully respect a person's decision in favor of comfort care? Or will we, perhaps without perceiving it, adopt a hint of the attitude the Pilgrim resident exhibited toward Marguerite?

2

Less-Traveled Paths

When it comes to imagining how to live with medical bad news, I venture that each of us "sees through a glass darkly." Learning that we or a loved one harbors a condition that portends a difficult future forces us at once to look inward and outward. But clarity in these moments and the months and years that follow may be difficult to achieve. One has to struggle to even know how to struggle. Though many people afflicted with serious or terminal diseases choose, like Marguerite, to be compliant with suggested treatments, even experimental ones, some decide to go their own way. What is it like to make one's own path? In this chapter I write about two people, one a young woman who was not ready to deal with her bad news and the other a physician colleague in his early forties who decided to make his own "playbook" for what he called his "final game."

DIANA AND DENIAL

One midweek morning in the late 1970s in San Francisco, a woman in her early twenties—big, strong, red hair going one way and scarves going the other—strode briskly into the ER demanding to be seen "Now!" When Diana got up that morning and was drinking coffee, she experienced blurred vision and a mild discomfort in her right eye. She had a job interview later that day, and she wanted a doctor to see her even though it was probably "just nerves." It had happened once before, a few months ago. Then it lasted "a few days" and went away. Probably nerves then, too, she said, as she was breaking up with her boyfriend at the time.

"Any other problems with your vision?"

"No."

"Any problems with any numbness or tingling in your arms or legs, anywhere in your body? Any problems with your balance, your movements?"

At first a "No" to all, but then a hesitation and "Yes, some numbness sometimes, in my right hand and my left leg. Not now, though."

"Any diseases? Now or previously? Any medicines, including eye drops, or recreational drugs?"

Again, "No" to all.

We could have run a lot of tests that morning, and eventually someone probably did, but a telling clue to Diana's puzzle lay in her routine physical exam. When I shined a light at her right pupil, instead of contracting, which is normal, it dilated slightly. When I looked through her pupils at the back of her eyes, I sensed that her right optic disk was slightly inflamed, though I was not sure. For Diana, a woman of Northern European extraction in her early twenties, these symptoms of blurred vision and numbness in different limbs at different times and the sign of her abnormal pupil response strongly suggested that she had early multiple sclerosis. MS is a disease of the central nervous system in which the coatings of the nerves degenerate unevenly. Although the disease invariably progresses and incapacitates those who have it, most people with MS experience an undulating course of symptom flare-ups followed by relative calm and eventual relapses. People with MS usually live for decades, and the disease course often gives them enough time to learn how to adapt to its impositions. Now, as then, medical science cannot predict the daily or weekly path of someone with MS.

When I finished my exam, I sat down and collected myself before speaking. Although I recall starting slowly—she was jumpy and I wanted us to be as calm as possible—it did not seem to make any difference. When I said that there might be a serious cause of her visual symptoms and past numbness, a physical problem in her nervous system, she got up and prepared to leave. I stayed seated. "Don't go just yet, Diana. Please hear me out. I cannot be sure of this, but you may be experiencing the very early stage of a disease called multiple sclerosis. It's a serious disease, and I'd like to call one of our neurologists to see you now if possible."

"Nooooooo!" she screamed. "Some other asshole ER doctor told me that once. You're wrong!" She ran out. I never saw her again, and she never called Neurology, at least not in the next year.

I saw Diana in the late 1970s. At that time, medical science had no test that proved one did or did not have MS. Nowadays, MRIs usually can make the diagnosis even early in the disease, but then all we had to go on were the patient's patterns of symptoms—her blurred vision and limb numbness—and signs, such as her pupil responses. We had tests, to be sure, but they were inconclusive.

Aside from our dramatic encounter, Diana's predicament has stayed with me. Suppose she had remained that morning and seen the neurologist, and suppose he confirmed my diagnosis and she had become a regular MS patient. Medicine in those days had few treatments to offer people with MS that would make their lives significantly better. Indeed, treatments that slow the course of the disease by a third or so only started appearing about ten years ago, and they work for many but not all patients. The other treatments that MS patients receive are not specific to MS; they aid in managing symptoms, such as loss of bladder control, that are common to many diseases.

Assuming that my diagnosis was correct, Diana had a real disease, one that likely has shortened her life and made it intermittently miserable. In those days, however, doctors could offer little beyond the reassurance of an ongoing relationship and some medicines of mild potency for particular problems. I speculate that subsequent episodes of alarming symptoms brought her back to other ERs and eventually into medicine's fold, but perhaps not.

Perhaps she chose to live in the wild, if you will, and not be domesticated. I had seen her in San Francisco, where, then and now, many with chronic illnesses choose to live outside medical orthodoxy. Her experiences, however distressing, would be hers—borne alone, perhaps, though one hopes not. She would be free from having her life "medicalized." It is a negative freedom, to be sure, but the "freedoms from" are important liberties nonetheless. In practical terms it would mean that her day-to-day life would be informed by what she chose to learn about her illness from friends, popular health texts, and nowadays the Internet. Visits to doctors—probably ER doctors—would be reserved for those episodes when things seemed to be out of control. Importantly, it would likely mean that her sense of time—*her* time, her existence—would differ qualitatively from what she would experience if she participated fully in the rituals of chronic medical care. For one thing, her life would be uncluttered by the endless medical visits, tests, and unrelenting treatments endured by people with serious chronic conditions.

If submitting to a medical regimen could do something real for her in terms of her own experience as much as in terms of her disease's course, then submission would seem wise. But what if medicine could not deliver that reality, as it could not in the 1970s for people with MS? What would her time be like then? Would her medical regime, with its requirements of attendance and obedience, take her out of her present? Would she feel she had become her disease long before the disease had achieved its imperium? Especially when the tests only monitored the disease and the treatments did little to alleviate and nothing to halt or cure, why should she go down the orthodox path? I never saw Diana again, so I do not know which path she chose. Had she accepted a follow-up appointment in Neurology but not shown up, or shown up once and then failed to appear for subsequent appointments, she would likely have been labeled, then as now, "noncompliant."

MIKE: A QUARTERBACK'S OUTSIDE RUN

Unlike Diana, Mike was too much a medical insider ever to be labeled as noncompliant. Though he enjoyed playing the role of gadfly in our medical center, he grew up as one of those who always knew they wanted to be a doctor. Teaching and practicing emergency medicine formed the core of his adult identity as intensely as playing quarterback in football had shaped his youth and college. A big, handsome, and muscular guy aware of the seductiveness of his charisma, he was used to shaping situations according to his vision. Most of the time this suited the common good, for Mike was smart and caring. He knew what it took to move a team down the field.

Mike reported nominally to me as departmental chair, though I doubt anyone ever controlled him. I did not find him particularly easy to work with, though our relationship was cordial enough. I was the one who had to deal with the administrative fallout of his gadfly activism. He was no fan of our new chancellor and made sure the chancellor knew it. Indeed, when I came aboard, the chancellor gave me carte blanche to remake the department, mentioning Mike by name. But I did not want to do that. I admired Mike's energy, if not always his style.

I am grateful I held back, for Mike and his wife Marge taught me a great lesson: what it is like to live on one's own terms with a terminal diagnosis. In telling what I know of Mike's story, I use my words and his. Doctors' accounts of their own struggles with terminal illnesses are rare, and rarer still are chronicles that attempt to see another from the outside in *and* the inside out. We are always and never quite what we seem to ourselves. About six months after I came to the Monarch of the Prairies Medical Center as a new departmental chair, Mike pulled me aside after a staff meeting to say he wanted to talk. We were working together on a grant for a new teaching program, but he said that wasn't the reason. What he wanted me to know was that he was about to go public with some personal news: he had just learned that he had esophageal cancer and that it had likely spread to his liver and maybe elsewhere.

I must have seemed startled, because immediately he said, "Yup, I couldn't believe it either. When I went last week to Abe, my doc in Family Practice, we both just figured this occasional discomfort I have here"—he pointed to his lower chest—"was a little reflux esophagitis from this hiatal hernia I've had forever. We even joked about cancer phobias and the waste of barium and X-ray film for my upper GI." What the upper GI showed, however, was barium flowing around an irregular mass at the border of Mike's esophagus and stomach. Two days later a colleague in GI put an endoscope down his throat and extracted a biopsy from his esophagus, which Pathology diagnosed to be a glandular cancer. Two days ago, Mike said, a CAT scan revealed a large solitary mass in his liver, presumably a metastasis, or spread of the cancer. Mike was forty-two then, and if well past his quarterbacking glory, he nonetheless still appeared to be a man in his physical prime. I expect that made the grisly news seem all the more unbelievable to him and probably also to his wife, Marge. After all, they had married just a few months ago.

For those who work in health care, such news can be especially poignant, as our training and experience gives us foreknowledge. Each of us has taken care of one or more individuals with a similar problem. In one sense this gives us an advantage—knowing what likely lies ahead, we tell ourselves that we will plan to deal with it in as rational a way as possible. Though we may first despair, we are primed to expect that we will remain in control—not of the disease, of course, but of our responses. Unlike the naive, who may be thrown off course for good by their new diagnosis, we assure ourselves that we will not lose our inner compass. First, of course, we must get a firm grasp of the possibilities.

For Mike, this meant an urgent consultation with the Monarch's senior oncologist, whom we both knew from our joint work on the Monarch's ethics committee. In that setting, she always came across as well prepared and empathic, quick to grasp the subtleties of the concerns of the affected parties. When Mike and Marge saw her, though, he told me afterward that they found her distant, that whatever concern she may have felt seemed obscured by her resort to the arcane language of survival rates and chemo protocols. I wasn't present, so I don't know what really happened. I do know that Mike was shaken, for I saw him later that day to let him know that he needn't worry about how long he was out, that we would make sure his obligations and salary were covered regardless. He listened, then switched the conversation back to the oncologist, saying almost in a mumble, "She seemed so cold. Info mode, no feeling. Surgery, she says, but nothing curative. Just palliative, just palliative." He said he and Marge would find someone else.

Since Mike's primary problem likely lay in his chest—no one would know for certain until the surgery and some additional tests—he and Marge next consulted our senior cardiothoracic surgeon, though not without initial misgivings. Whereas the oncologist was known, at least in her committee work, for her informed empathy, the surgeon, also a woman, was known for her brusque manner in the day-to-day world of the operating room, consultations, and hospital committees. Indeed, she and Mike, who also could be brusque, had traded cold words on a few occasions.

But in medicine, as in so much else in life, what one sees on someone's surface is not always what one gets. When medical students first approach patients to learn how to conduct medical interviews, they often assume they need to adopt a variant of the warm and avuncular manner of some imagined all-purpose healer. But many of them say being "warm and fuzzy" feels alien to them. After all, they prevailed in their premedical courses, sometimes ruthlessly, by being thinkers first and feelers second. (As one might expect, sitting in on students' early interviews with patients, like listening to bad karaoke, can make for a long afternoon.) Those of us who have been around longer know that what really counts with patients is the ability to convey to them that they have one's full attention. What encourages us as teachers is that we have learned we can teach almost any student who is willing that a connection with patients can be established if you are willing to learn how to listen actively.

It does not surprise me that the great surgeons I have known, whatever their outward manner, tend to have fanatically loyal patients. However economical of word and gesture they may be, they communicate what needs to be conveyed by a doctor toward patients: recognition of their plight and assurance that he will attend to them with his full capabilities. Of course, Mike knew this, too. When his surgeon recommended an aggressive approach, what she called by turns a "curative resection" and "radical cancer surgery," he and Marge went for it, though they knew the odds for its being "curative" were slight. What cemented their relationship with this person—so newly important in Mike's life—was her call to them on the Sunday before Mike's operation to see how they were doing. She talked with them, Mike later told me, as if she had all the time in the world, which touched him and Marge.

Even so, his hospital experience—massive surgery, three days in the ICU, chest tubes in, ventilator, intravenous pumps that worked for a while and then failed, excruciating pain, and so on—was, as is the case with so many, a nightmare. I know he never forgave the surgical resident who denied him morphine before taking out his chest tubes.

Mike stayed home for the next two months to recover, and though we talked weekly, I only saw him once in those weeks. The news from Pathology was worse than he expected: not only was the liver mass a metastasis from the esophageal tumor, but his regional lymph nodes also contained cancer. By definition, he was in Stage IV. The experts he talked with—and he reached back to his contacts from his residency days in New York City as well as to those at the Monarch—all said the same thing: no treatment from here on out was likely to alter his cancer's course.

In those early months after his operation, Mike told me he had no idea one could suffer so much. The stabbing pain in his chest wall from the surgery was overwhelming. When he tried to eat, he could not, as the stricture from the surgical manipulation of his esophagus and stomach caused him to "dump food" regularly and painfully. His children—two boys in their teens from his previous marriage—could barely stand to be around him. He could barely stand to look at or be with himself, he said. His grief was too intense. In six weeks he lost forty pounds. Marge was hanging in there, he said. "She's great. Unbelievable!" But even she could cry with him only so much, and he said he often cried alone while she slept.

What I saw when I visited him at home was a man who looked ravaged in every way. He then expected, because his doctors had told him so, that he would live only about six months more. That was why, he told me, he wanted to go so deeply into his grief. Catholic by upbringing and nominally observant as an adult, Mike said he needed to keep going into "the silence," that he felt it was the best way to prepare himself and his family for what lay ahead. I have known other terminally ill people whose spiritual quest took a mystical turn. Because he had conducted so much of his previous life as part of a team, I thought he might reconnect with his church contacts as he went inward, but he said no, not then. He did have a group of tight friends, all men, from diverse backgrounds. Every few months they made a point of gathering at a special place out on the prairie and talking about their lives, and he looked forward to getting together with them soon. But for now it was just Marge and he and his kids going it alone. He just wanted enough time to "get ready to die." That must have been the low point for Mike.

When I saw him next, three months had elapsed since his surgery. Though still thin and looking as though he had experienced prolonged physical stress, Mike nonetheless seemed immeasurably better. He wanted to come back to work, "half-time if possible," he said, and "no nights, if that's OK." Yes, he was sure he was ready. No, he did not want to be double-covered, which means that another one of us staff physicians would work with him in case fatigue set in suddenly. But I insisted.

"All right. Try your damn double coverage, at least for a couple of shifts." Yes, it seemed the old Mike was reemerging.

I asked him what had changed.

"What has changed, Dear Leader," he smiled, "is that I am free!"

"This is great news!" I said. "What's going on?"

Mike responded that nothing had changed and everything had changed. He wasn't sure how it had come about, but his grief was gone. Once he was able to get up and around easily, he and Marge arranged to see another oncologist for a second opinion. What his new doctor suggested, Mike continued, was that he use his fore-knowledge to free himself from "the system."

When Mike initially protested to his doctor that medical insight into the future wouldn't change anything and that he was soon to die, the oncologist countered that his departure was not that imminent. Could Mike not see that he was in fact gaining weight; that his aggressive surgery, which had included removal of part of his liver, was likely to have gained him considerable time? If so, then why not choose to live? Don't bother with Phase II trials and repeat CAT scans to follow the "progress" of the cancer, Mike paraphrased the oncologist. *We* know they won't make any difference. When the time comes, we will arrange the best hospice care possible.

Mike said he walked out of that meeting feeling as if a great weight had been lifted off his shoulders. My hunch was that this physician's approval of a laissez-faire approach was the catalyst Mike needed to regain his sense of self. The cancer was in him, to be sure, but he was not yet "cancerous Mike." Instead, he remained a Mike who happened to have a serious cancer. Yes, he had pain—the pain from his thoracotomy dogged him to the end—and yes, he could only eat small amounts of food at one time, but if he claimed it, he still had considerable room to make his own life. That a specialist in cancer had said so was all Mike needed to take over the ball. As with so much else in his life, he could be in the system and tweak it to serve his purposes. "Nothing" had suddenly become "everything."

As we talked and I felt his happiness, I remembered Marguerite and Eduardo and wondered what they would have done, given the same opportunity. During the next year, Mike gradually returned to working almost full-time. Though we had to cover his shifts without additional staffing, none of us begrudged him this. We were happy to see him happy. Since he did not expect to live that long, he and Marge decided to indulge themselves with a few splurges. Nothing too elaborate—a remodeled kitchen and a delayed honeymoon to Italy were the extent of it, I think. He told me he had tidied up his domestic "loose ends," by which he meant devising a living will, and educational trusts for his boys. Around the middle of that year, Mike, who had a fondness for dramatic flourishes, started talking with me and others about how living with a terminal illness added "light" to his life. "Living with the Angel of Death on my shoulder," he called it, and he gave a moving talk to the medical students about his new experiences. He spoke of what it meant for him now to be "radically honest" with everyone. The medical students, obliged to nod endlessly to whatever any senior person said to them, from the interns on up, loved that bit. He also talked about how important for him it had become to nourish his relationships with others. Sometimes this meant reconnecting with past friends; mostly it meant a new intensity of feeling for his wife and family. He did not acknowledge that his new freedom had a shadowy side; perhaps he did not see it. We did: he flung increasingly pointed insults at the upper administration, and a few more declarations of "Fuck this!" came out in his activist pep talks with the students. As one would expect, the complaints often came my way, but they remained manageable.

In the middle of the following year—his second "above ground," as Mike liked to say—we in the ER began to notice a change. Gradually, he seemed to withdraw emotionally from us. Though his physical condition remained more or less the same, he no longer wanted to join us for after-work outings and began to shy away from any encounters not related to the patients he was seeing that day. I have seen this happen with other people with terminal diagnoses. I had many patients and several friends with HIV in San Francisco during the 1980s. Those were the days before treatments existed to control the virus. Even so, some patients and friends then lived for a long time between learning they were HIV positive and developing the various complications of AIDS. Over time, though, they tended to withdraw into themselves. The few who talked with me about it said they felt "marked," that they knew they could "never go back." For them, their illness would always be in the foreground. Because it was, they felt a new kinship with the dying, and felt that their capacity for friendship with the uninfected, the adamantly living, was dwindling. Again, it was not because they felt ill, for they mostly did not. It was because death was a part of their future in a way that it never seems to be for those not afflicted with a terminal diagnosis.

For my part, I began to experience with Mike what I had experienced with them: weariness with his foreground, which in its abbreviated form consisted of his oft-repeated "living with the Angel." With him, as I had with them, I felt crowded out by his diagnosis. Mike's sons later told me that they had experienced a gradual loss of emotional traction with him, too. For them, of course, this had a more personal import: they felt they "couldn't reach" their dad anymore, at least not as they had. At first they felt guilty. I expect he did, too, though he did not speak of it with me. I do not know how Marge felt.

Although such relational slippages are strange and uncomfortable for those obliged to stretch across their gaps, they occur routinely in families or friendships in which one member is living with a fatal disease. Long-dormant springs of guilt often resume bubbling as well. Indeed, families with a terminally ill member often fracture. Even when the affected person functions almost normally, the centrifugal force of their new sense of mortality may pull them out to the fringe of their group and beyond. A few end up alone. Mike's family seemed to have handled his sense of foreboding rather well, which could not have been easy. For all Mike's talk of Marge as his "equal partner in everything," from what I could tell, their family functioned as a patriarchy. He spoke and they listened, a habit that probably made the whole process more tolerable than it would have been otherwise. When his sons decided to spend more time at their mother's, fortunately he did not shame them or protest; paradoxically, he seemed to demonstrate more interest in them.

Mike's life during his next year, his third after learning he was ill with advanced cancer, took another spiritual turn. I first noted it when he made what seemed like an odd request. Knowing of my training in history, he asked me what I knew of the history of death. What he wanted to know about in particular was the history of images of death, like the dancing skeletons that figured in Renaissance imaginations. Did I know where he could find some? He wanted, he said, to get in touch with his "inner skeleton," his "sense of rot." I did not know much about the subject, but I was able to locate some texts and images for him. They seemed to serve him as talismans. As he put it one afternoon in his office, they helped him see that God and death "are cut from the same cloth." Gradually, photocopies of old German Dances of Death replaced some of the political activist slogans that had previously papered his office walls. Around this time he started wearing a black leather trench coat. He also started to return to church, not the Catholic Church of his Irish origins, but a vibrant Baptist congregation that gathered in a black neighborhood.

Mike was always clear with us that he entertained no hope of a "cure" for his illness. Indeed, what he emphasized to anyone who would listen was that he had a lot of hope and that he kept it focused on his day-to-day life. Reluctant to call himself a "cancer survivor," he chose instead to say he was a person who had cancer. Usually he followed this with an invocation of his "living with the Angel of Death on my shoulder" imagery. Though the phrase evoked for me the kitsch of a Precious Moments figurine, I sensed his rhetorical ornament helped keep him focused. In the ER, the nurses noticed he no longer wore a watch.

Mike also shifted his professional attention from our emergency medicine research projects to the nascent subspecialty of palliative care. Indeed, he became active at the Monarch in establishing a well-trained palliative care team, gave lectures on the subject, and participated in the national hospice movement. He seemed driven in this, often staying late to work on his new project. Living with advanced cancer made him newly aware of the importance of hospice, he said, and he was determined to make sure he remained "in control" of the end of *his* life. Early one evening I stopped by his office just to catch up and learned by chance how important this new work had become. He motioned me to sit down while he finished an e-mail to someone on his "cancer list" who needed an urgent reply. Intrigued, I waited until he finished and asked him to say more.

Maybe two months before, he said, he had taken up the suggestion of another person with esophageal cancer he met through his oncologist. Almost every cancer had its corresponding Internet group of affected persons and families, she told him. Why didn't he see what they were up to? It might help him feel more connected. "Haven't you been saying that the people around you don't know quite how to act about your illness? The group for esophageal cancer is very informal. Just share what's on your mind, where your fears are carrying you. You can make it anonymous or not. You're a doc; we'd all welcome someone with your knowledge and insights. Try out the group."

And so Mike began. Every two or three days, he said, he spent a few hours online with his group. He said it was changing his life. "Sharing my illness," he told me later, "helps me incredibly. I wish I knew why. I don't, but I can feel the effects of reaching out." I asked him if I could check out the site and follow along. Later, he gave me permission to share his interchanges with others. In what follows, I offer some of Mike's comments. Here are paraphrases of his e-mails:

May 2, 2000. Subject: First post. Greetings and salutations. My name is Mike Murphy. I live with my wife Marge and, on weekends, my two sons, who are now 15 and 17, from my previous marriage. I was a healthy 42 year old guy when I learned I had Stage IV adenocarcinoma with extension into adjacent structures— pls bear with the medspeak—local lymph nodes, and a solitary mass in my liver. My surgeon and I determined that my disease cannot be cured, so we decided to remove as much evidence of it as we could—what we called "radical palliative surgery"—to give me the most time possible. Afterward, I consulted lots of cancer specialists all over the U.S.—I'm a doctor in a medical school and so know quite a few. After listening to them, I decided that there was no good evidence that any additional cancer treatment would change how much time I have. So I have not had any cancer treatments since my surgery. That was a little over three years ago . . . Since then, I've been living the richest period of my life . . .

Enough about me for now. I join you to find good company and in order to share some of the wonderful things I've learned about living with cancer. For the past few months I've retooled my medical career in the direction of studying and teaching and providing palliative/hospice care. It's the area where I can best be a doc now. (I'm an ER doc by training and still work some shifts there.)

May 15, 2000. Response to post by Ralph: Ralph writes that his wife Betty died in four months because "she never thought she could win. Her doctor left her with no hope." I was given the same prognosis as Betty. Then I just wanted to get my affairs in order and arrange the most comfortable death I could. What we choose to make of our prognosis is critical. Hope for a "cure" is not the only kind of hope. For most of us with metastatic solid tumor cancers, hope for a cure is beyond our reach. But I do not lead a hopeless life. Some of us are leading lives more free and more full than we ever thought possible.

May 18, 2000. Response to post by Kathy re her dad's "struggle with mortality": When we deal with a life-threatening and usually terminal condition, we must do INTENSE GRIEF WORK. I cannot tell you enough how hard this is. Planning one's own funeral is just one of many experiences of extreme sadness I've been going through. Living with an illness like ours has immense psychological and spiritual dimensions along with the medical. We have to come to terms with our own mortality. At least this has been my biggest struggle. But deciding to live as fully as I can in this "*last game*" *of my life—I used to play football—has been spiritually enriching beyond what I thought possible. It's also been smart in a strategic sense because I can focus without guilt on what's important. I've discovered that being "terminal" is not really all that different from being "mortal."*

Once I got through the grief about my fate, which took a long time, I found my biggest problem in that struggle has been that I am attempting to change in a SOCIETY that does not want to talk about MORTALITY and DEATH! So my biggest day-to-day issue—and I'm curious about your dad's—is my increasing sense of isolation. Because I've told people I have metastatic cancer, I am "marked." Outside of my wife and sons, I hardly have any social life left. Yes, I go to work and have lots of work "friends," but they seem increasingly unwilling to get close to the skeleton inside me. So we pretend I'm the same old Mike. Except I'm not. Has anyone else been experiencing this?

So who do I go to for support in this area of living with cancer? I have a wonderful wife and sons, but they don't really want to hear about it. Luckily, I found out about a grade school buddy who has advanced cancer and lives elsewhere. We post each other a couple of times a week. I know some of you go to support groups regularly, but I haven't for over a year. It's been just my old buddy and me.

July 2, 2000. Re: end-of-life stuff. I want to be clear about what "hope" has come to mean for me. Many of us have hope in the Ultimate Source of our existence, and no medical prognosis can take away that kind of hope. There is also a kind of "natural hope," which I think is more like the hope for the best possible outcome, come whatever. And for people with both kinds of hope, talking about metastatic cancer only as a "battle" or "war" can get beside

the point. For some people the "battle" approach gives them hope.
But for some of us, planning for hospice care early, though we don't
need it now, does not extinguish our hope. After all, someone wins
the lottery . . . I happen to think that no specifically targeted can-
cer treatment will help me live longer or much better, so I am not
bothering with any. But then I've been lucky—I expected to die
about three years ago and am still going pretty strong.

I'm working in hospice because I've seen all too many dying
people come to it at the very end. Right now only about 15% of
dying Americans ever get hospice care, and a third of those start in
the last week of their lives. In the meantime, what do they think
they are doing—getting cured? Dying happens to each of us, yet
medicine has no diagnosis for it—no diagnostic code. Doesn't that
seem odd? Advanced cancers of all kinds are truly horrible diseases,
but they have one slight advantage compared to other bad diseases
like heart disease, Alzheimer's, etc., and that is this: Cancer usu-
ally follows a predictable downward course. Usually it gives us time
to come to terms with our inevitable oblivion. That's why hospice
began in relation to caring for people with cancer—the disease gave
them time. Had I not had this disease, I am too much of the "hard
charger" type of person to ever have thought about my life as deeply
as I do now knowing that it will end. This awareness has been
a GIFT.

Alice wrote about her Bill: "Never in a million years would I
have let someone else take care of him in hospice." But in America
right now over 90% of hospice happens in the dying person's
HOME, with the care provided by family members, volunteers,
and teams of hospice consultants. In short, in hospice you have bet-
ter contact with your loved ones, not less.

August 15, 2000. Re: reply to Janice about my approach to cancer treatment. I'm sorry if my statements about treatments seem cruel. What I said was if a person has advanced cancer AND in spite of aggressive treatments (surgery, radiation & chemo) develops recurrent disease, then continued pursuit of aggressive treatments against "THE BEAST" is not the only way to go. There are several ways of living and dying with this disease, including what I've chosen—let's call it "comprehensive supportive care."

November 20, 2000. Re: a Very Sensitive Topic. So far I've tried to "pay my dues" to the group. It's been great responding to specific medical queries online and off line on the phone. Now I could use some help. My wife Marge and I had only been married a few months when I learned I had esophageal cancer. Our sex life had been GREAT!! But not great or even good for some time now though it's wonderful in every other way. She says it's because I seem to be focused on death—she just finds it hard to get interested in sex with me. I've looked in the literature but can't find anything out on this. If anyone has insight/resources on what happens to the partner without cancer re libido, PLS let me know.

March 20, 2001. Dear Group: Looks like my "time out" from the disease is over and I'm in the "endgame." I've been noticing hoarseness and having headaches. It turns out that mets in my lungs and brain are the cause. The docs—surgeons—want to "take 'em out," but Marge and I are not sure. I know I won't let them open my chest again—I cannot go through that twice in this life. I am losing my voice, which is a drag . . . I know I don't want chemo for the masses in my chest—from what I can tell, chemo used in a "palliative" way just hasn't worked in solid tumors, especially in slow-growing ones like mine.

It's freaky—I'm writing this having just swallowed prednisone pills to shrink the cancer in my brain so I can write about cancer in my brain. But I'm doing it so I can also hear the Voice of God, which comes through with increasing ease.

March 27, 2001. Well, I decided to let the neurosurgeons/radiotherapists "ZAP" the lesion in my brain. They say it all went very well. My headaches are gone, but I'm very tired. Now to rest up and see about my voice.

April 4, 2001. Good and bad news about my voice—but isn't that usually the case with doctors?! My left vocal cord is totally paralyzed because my main tumor is eroding the nerve that controls it. Can't fix that . . . Have been weeping a lot—grieving for my voice. In my "endgame," it would help me to know that we had rituals in this country to remember our dead, something like the Mexican "Dia de los Muertos." I'm talking with my family about keeping up a "vital connection" with them, but I fear it "creeps out" my sons, especially the younger one, who is now almost 16. Marge has been great. She has no problem when I let her know how scared I am. Lots of pain from the masses in my chest. Have started on narcotic skin patches, which help.

May 24, 2001. A new complication on the field: about 2 weeks ago I started to have MUCHO MAS pain in my back and left shoulder. Well, it turns out the tumor is going through one of my upper spinal column bones and into my spinal cord. No wonder the narcotics don't work. I changed my earlier decision about "no treat-

ment" and decided to go with a course of 10 radiations to shrink the mass and gain relief. So far have had 4. I can hardly move or even read . . .

June 12, 2001. Wish I hadn't allowed myself to get sucked into the cancer patient role—the treatments for my back didn't work. Have signed up as a patient on our new Palliative Care Service. Of course, they're taking good care of me on my visits—I helped set up the team! I wish I were 75 when this was happening to me and not 45, but in a sense each of us needs a disease to experience a good death. Cancer ain't bad in this regard, for its course is fairly predictable. It has given me the three best years of my life and time to arrange a meaningful passage from this world . . .

My younger son won't talk about my situation at all.

Re: Stewart's question about hydration/nutrition for his dad: People not familiar with what the body goes through in dying assume that dehydration and malnutrition are painful or involve serious suffering. For those dying from intestinal cancers, stopping eating is a relief. Pain control should stay aggressive, but studies from hospice show that stopping fluids does NOT seem to cause suffering.

August 20, 2001. I am unofficially leaving the group. I've closed my office and come home to my porch and bedroom to die . . . I've been working on a set of scrapbooks with my boys and it has let us be together in ways that don't frighten them so much. Physically, things gradually worsen, with supplemental oxygen at night now. Marge and I speculate on how we will maintain some relationship after I die. Who knows? I do hope she meets a great guy when she's ready. Yes, I hope she remarries—I can't see her being a widow for

*the rest of her life. She's really been extraordinary. Thank you all
for everything. Peace, Mike.*

Mike died on September 15, 2001, at home in the company of
his wife and sons. Though he may not have remained in as complete control of his final stages as he had hoped, he came pretty
close. His advocacy for living richly in the light and shadows of
death also helped move his team a good bit down the field of life's
final possibilities, to use his phrasing. I think Mike would have loved
his funeral. More than five hundred people packed his church,
which stood in the middle of a public housing project. Many spoke
about him; the service lasted for more than three hours. Lots of
singing and call and response. I sat next to the chancellor. About
halfway through the service he whispered to me, "So how long
does it take to bury this guy? My driver's waiting." By the third
hour he couldn't stop fidgeting. Had Mike been there to notice, I
expect he would have smiled.

3

Illusions of Control

How should one approach the big decisions in life? In health and sickness, Mike Murphy assumed that "being in control" was the best way to be, and most of us probably would agree. The more we are in control, we tell ourselves, the better our lives will be, the freer we will be. "I feel so *empowered*, so much more in *control*, so *free* . . ." We say this inwardly and to each other, many of our parents say it up into their seventies, and our teenage children say it, or versions of it, all the time. Even when I find expressions of the foregoing ludicrous, I nonetheless live and move through my world as if it were so, as if achievement of power and control were a goal with deep worth. And so does almost everyone else I know, especially those who work in medicine and those with life-threatening medical problems who seek us out. Achievement of control has taken on the status of a moral and aesthetic imperative. It suffuses our relationships, our machines, our politics, our approach to nature, and, for those of us who are religious, perhaps our theology. Yet an old definition for the English words *patient* and *patience* is "willingness to endure, even to endure suffering," phrases that suggest the value of resilience without implying a need to dominate.

It may come as a surprise to realize just how recently preoccupation with power and control has moved to the foreground of medical care. Indeed, aside from vaccines and a few antibiotics and hormones to control infections and metabolic derangements like high blood sugar, the idea that anyone could control desperate *medical* conditions has only arisen since World War II. As late as the 1950s, the way doctors cared for patients with heart attacks, for example, was closer to the year 1 C.E. than to today, as the following description of a scene from a 1950 Manhattan hospital film suggests.

When a middle-aged man clutches his chest and slumps to the street, presumably from a heart attack, his companion phones the hospital. Next we see an intern, alerted in his call room, stubbing out his cigarette and running to the ambulance. Sirens wail through midtown traffic. The young doc arrives on the scene and places an oxygen mask on the afflicted. So far, so good. When they reach the ER, though, the intern takes the oxygen mask off and everyone waits for the patient's "regular doctor" to arrive. The nurse gives the patient an injection of morphine in the interim, but that is about it. And what happens when the patient's regular physician arrives? An exam, EKG, X-rays, and a blood draw for tests, to be sure, and then upstairs to a regular room for bed rest.

That was advanced care in those days—no ICUs, few machines, relatively few medicines, the rare IV, and little understanding of the pathophysiology of heart attacks. Doctors did not expect to "control" the outcomes of these unstable situations, and their patients did not expect them to. Doctors and nurses could sincerely tell their patients they were doing everything they could, in part because they could do so little. When therapeutic modesty gave way to widespread new enthusiasm for technologies of bodily control that began in the mid-1960s and took off in the 1970s, the older way did not linger for long. Indeed, other than prompt administration of oxygen, about the only similarity between critical care then and now is that ambulances still take almost as long to cross midtown Manhattan as they did in 1890, let alone 1950.

Those of us who have been living through these decades have celebrated the disappearance of therapeutic modesty, or rather the arrival of its aggressive successors, as the triumph of high-tech medicine. Not only do we expect ever more from our medical machines and drugs, we doctors also expect to be more in control of ourselves. In the Pilgrim ER, for instance, at one point we monitored, minute by minute, the correctness and timing of our interventions on people arriving with possible heart attacks. By the end of the study, we had cut our average time from arrival to initiation of definitive treatment from what it had been—around seventy-five minutes, which is not good—to twenty-five minutes, which put us among the best. Control means little without ongoing surveillance.

In the meantime, "empowerment" and "being in control" have transformed older ethical norms of how doctors and patients ought to behave with each other. The paternalism of the Hippocratics and Marcus Welby, M.D.—"Doctor knows best"—has been discredited in favor of models that privilege a patient's autonomy. Some ethicists and many corporations maintain that "patients" have really turned into "customers" for "health care products and services." A person who shops for the best deal for a Lasik lens correction or a nose job, like the doctor advertising the deal, might as well go with such a customer model. (Not so, perhaps, for the victim of a gunshot wound to the chest who needs an emergent chest tube to survive. Assuming he did not shoot himself, discussion of his autonomy is rather beside the point, at least in the ER.) Other new ethical models retain the "patients" as such, but now they are patients who are to participate proactively or "contract with" their doctors. HMOs and some neocon ethicists like these models, and so do many patients—at least until they experience a denial of coverage from their insurance plan.

What each one of these models shares is the assumption that respect for the patient's autonomy trumps other considerations. For reasonable adults who desire to be "in control," this assumption makes eminent sense. Through the medium of the vernacular medical bibles of Google and Yahoo, it is also achievable. In essence, that is how Mike Murphy chose to live with his illness. With a sensibility that echoes the strict individualism of the Protestant Reformation, newly savvy patients who pursue this path are reacting to traditional medical assertions of authority—Trust us, we always know more! This recalls early struggles between Bible-clutching Lutherans and their opponents, Catholic authorities who preferred to retain control of sacred knowledge and the authority that comes with monopoly. As one might expect, many senior medical leaders are not enthusiastic about their newly restive patients—not in private, anyway.

Medicine's cultural sea change—the profession and public's new infatuation with control and power and its shadow, a crisis of professional authority—may seem like the weather, an impersonal set of forces to which one tries to adapt. But for people with critical illnesses, this is hardly the case. Adaptation is not always possible, and the forces are not impersonal. Nowhere in medicine is this more apparent than in the spaces where the very sick spend their time—the high-tech ICUs that proliferate in our hospitals and their mini-ICU counterparts in some of our ERs. Although many critically ill people enter ICUs only to emerge days or weeks later with a new lease on life, many suffer needlessly during and after their stay or die in needlessly prolonged misery while there. What began as utopia of sorts in the 1960s and 1970s has become, for many, dystopia in the 2000s.

How and why does this happen? Why do intense hospital experiences leave so many feeling fractured or worse? No simple answer suffices, and many specialists in critical care are studying a host of contributory technical factors. Instead of summarizing the current state of knowledge, this chapter includes two brief stories that illustrate what may be our general tendency—and that of the machines and spaces we have created—to imagine our desired realities in terms of power and control. In the quotidian of ICU life, the paradox is that instead of enhancing and preserving us, these frameworks often macerate our humanity and sometimes our very lives. But it does not need to be this way. I write this chapter as by turns a witness, a modest reformer, and, for those about to endure a spate of ICU life, a guide.

YES, YOU CAN BE TOO RICH

In comparison with any populous society in recorded history or our foreign contemporaries today—or ourselves in 1961—in America we publicly celebrate *having* as the most important dimension of human experience. *Having* operates in several realms, not least a tendency to organize one's existence around acquiring things, the most tangible aspect of our consumer society. But the compulsion to experience life as a process of having extends deeper and wider into areas at once abstract and personal. Not only do we have a sense of our bodies as something we *own*, as compared to living marvels we *inhabit*, as patients we feel a sense of entitlement to unlimited medical treatments, and as physicians to provide them, regardless. We imagine we *possess* life, that we own our bodies and minds, and that if something goes wrong, we will have procedures or pills or new parts that will fix our property. Though we know otherwise, still we behave as if all this that we have—our bodies, minds, stuff, others—will extend horizontally to an indefinite horizon, with death lying just beyond sight.

Increasingly, Americans even approach religion, an area that traditionally offers refuge from a preoccupation with having, as another means of getting more in material terms, at least as measured by the growth of sects that advertise a gift for achieving earthly "success" for their members. Contrary to the intentions of the founding figures of most major religions, our temples are full of sellers and buyers.

Forty years ago, phrases such as *health science campuses*, *the health care industry*, and the ubiquitous new dyad of *health care consumer* and *health care provider* did not exist. These rhetorical moves may be subtle, but they signal a deep shift: the commodification of something that resists being turned into a commodity, which is health. The old "medicine," in comparison, at least recognized its boundaries.

We doctors treat disease, and often, if the disease, our current knowledge, and expertise permit, the disease goes away or into remission. Just as often, perhaps, the disease goes away of its own accord. In either situation, the absence of disease permits a person to return to her usual state of health. We may also be able to repair a defect—a cleft lip, say—that is not a disease but nonetheless inhibits a full life. But we engage in existential sleight of hand if we pretend that treating diseases equates to delivering or even understanding health as most people experience it in everyday life.

We—doctors and patients alike—confuse ourselves if we assume that biomedicine (and the corporate interests that increasingly shape its imagination) can and should tell us the purpose and meaning of our lives. *That* existential terrain belongs to notions of wholeness, integrity, and being, ancient concepts that encompass both a sense of surrender to the fact of our own existence and unsentimental embrace of that existence. Whatever treatment advances and bodily insights biotechnology and the life sciences may generate, I believe they remain by their very nature unable to capture *health*, though they may make it possible. When they cannot cure or prevent, as by definition they cannot with chronic afflictions, they still may alleviate suffering.

Just under the surface of our infatuation with power and control—clearly visible, not even lurking—is the American celebration of individual wealth. In the new oligarchy that has arisen since the 1970s, it is as though one can never have too much, as though the ability of wealth to manipulate circumstances is a form of power to be enacted above all others. If this were so, then one would assume that very rich people receive the best of care. In my experience, however, this has not been the general case. Granted, they often enjoy the most attentive care, especially from senior staff, but the ability of wealth to control circumstances only extends so far into one's body. In the meantime, the golden aura that sur-rounds the very rich often blinds them and those around them to the value of ordinary common sense.

Successful by birthright in what she jokingly referred to as "the inheritance business," Betsy, who was known for being charm-ing and imperious by turns, married Richard the week after she graduated from college. Though they fought about who was "in charge" during their early years, the tensions eased as the clever Richard made a fortune on his own in Silicon Valley. By their early fifties, Betsy and Richard had decided to trade entrepreneurial ad-venturing for more time with each other, their friends, and the grandchildren two of their four sons and their wives were begin-ning to produce. All but one of the sons lived nearby, which meant they routinely got together at one or another's house or at the family ranch above Carmel. Betsy even started to cook—a de-velopment that astonished her husband and sons.

When Richard's jet crashed in a Montana fog on his way back from a fishing trip during his fifty-ninth summer, everything changed. Even after the first year of his absence, Betsy seemed to her friends still lost in deep grief. When she went out to a board meeting or a grandchild's birthday party, the engagement hardly seemed to matter: a few smiles and easy words, and then the hol-low eyes of someone without much hope. It was a pity she was not religious, her friends said. *Carpe diem* had been her and Richard's motto. While he was alive, it worked well for them, but not now. Only her youngest, aged twenty-three and still at home, realized that Betsy had begun drinking secretly and heavily. Lost in a funk of his own, compounded by his fondness for cocaine, he made only a halfhearted effort at confronting her. Richard had been her ballast. Now that he was gone, she could not seem to find her balance. She knew it and complained about it, but that did not mean she was going to listen to anybody else, including her son. Her house staff knew, of course, but though they had been with her family for years, they were not about to take up her drinking with her. Even when Betsy's youngest alerted her doctor, she easily placated the latter with a promise to go light on the booze and fill his trial prescription for an antidepressant. Everyone hoped she would soon feel better.

As with many querulous drunks with money—*querulous drunk* is an infelicitous phrase, true, but alcoholism degrades everyone it touches—Betsy's worst tendencies increasingly took over. Frustrated by her bossiness and catty remarks, old friends from her girlhood called less. When her chronic bronchitis turned into "walking pneumonia," she tossed off her physician's advice to enter the hospital. Why go into the hospital, she asked him rhetorically, when I have an excellent staff at home? "My butler will arrange for some nurses, and you can prescribe the antibiotics." Cowed, he did not push the point, and Betsy remained at home.

But germs have a life of their own, and as time passed Betsy's morbid ones made their way from her lungs into her bloodstream and then her meninges, the coverings of her brain. When her butler finally brought her to the ER, she was in a stupor, with a high fever and headache. Her exam and tests confirmed that she was experiencing bacterial meningitis. For the first couple of days, the ICU staff thought they detected improvement. Her fever went down, and the stupor of her initial presentation seemed a little lighter. Even so, her children became more worried. Though long estranged from his mother and late father, her eldest son returned home from London to set up a "command post" for their extensive network. A couple of weeks passed, and by the end of them Betsy seemed only minimally conscious. Once or twice she seemed a little "better," responding, perhaps purposely, to some stimuli—a groan when a catheter was changed, for example—but she did not wake up.

Before she became ill, Betsy had made it clear in writing to her sons and regular physician and lawyer that she did not want to live "like a vegetable." But then who determines when someone becomes "a vegetable" and when someone's wishes should be honored? Pressed by her sons for their opinion, her doctors—and she had quite a team—could not initially agree. Her eldest son, citing "Mom's wishes," said he did not want to "drag it out." But no one quite trusted him. Did he not come to her ICU bed from the airport with a well-thumbed copy of Betsy's will in his carry-on? Although things did not look good, was he not crossing the line by talking at night with his brothers about how to divide things up? Betsy's youngest, for one, was not ready to let go. The oldest, using guilt—"You were around, why didn't you do something sooner, you pathetic cokehead!"—shamed the youngest. But the youngest held out for more time. As so often happens in critical illness, the family, the whole focus of Betsy's life, threatened to fall apart.

Even though Betsy sank ever more deeply into coma, the ICU's chief neurologist continued to report that she was doing "well" or, if she made some reflexive twitch, that she was doing "better." The brothers quarreled, weeks passed, and Betsy's condition did not change. Finally, her lawyer, a longtime family friend, persuaded the sons to find out exactly what the ICU chief meant by "better." Through talking with the nurses, they learned that this physician was notorious for insisting, "No one ever dies on my service, not if I can help it!" At that point Betsy's lawyer obtained a second neurological opinion. When the second expert determined that Betsy would never recover any significant function, her children, though no longer talking with each other, agreed through their mother's lawyer to stop the full-court press. When her next infection came, her eldest son exercised his legal surrogacy not to initiate additional treatment, and Betsy died shortly thereafter. Within a year, her youngest son died accidentally from a drug overdose.

Betsy's initial refusal to enter the hospital for definitive care of her pneumonia, which is probably what enabled her infection to establish itself thoroughly in her meninges while she was still at home, may have sealed her fate. But would things have gone differently for her and her children, would she have avoided the degradation of an extended demise and they a catastrophic rupture, if her ICU doctors, especially her first neurologist, had reached agreement earlier on her prognosis? One cannot know for sure, but probably they would have. After all,when well, she had been clear about how she wanted to be cared for if she became permanently incapacitated. Had Betsy's medical team provided a univocal assessment of her situation, her sons, though divided, might have been able to come together in grief as they respected her wishes and let their mother go. Instead, as often happens when family members quarrel around the bed of a member who has entered death's penumbra, division among the doctors amplified preexisting division in the family. Procrastination for both groups set in, with the result that the single tragedy of the loss of a parent doubled itself in the loss of a son as well as any sense of family for her survivors.

MEDICAL FUTILITY
AND THE PROCESS OF DYING

For the past fifteen years or so, many physicians and bioethicists have devoted themselves to the conundrum at the heart of Betsy's final two months. According to them—and there have been several high-level conferences and commissions on the subject—the issue is one of determining when medical care becomes "futile." At first glance, determining "medical futility," as the circumstance has become known within medicine, seems straightforward: medically futile interventions are those that will not permit restoration of vital bodily functions in sustainable ways. A clear-cut example is the futility of performing an emergency thoracotomy—"cracking the chest"—on people who demonstrate no signs of life in the field because they have suffered massive blunt trauma to the chest in a motor vehicle collision. The chest can be opened when they are brought to an ER, but if they have experienced that form of injury and arrive at its doors with no signs of life, numerous outcome studies demonstrate that no intervention will "bring them back."

However, as Betsy's situation suggests, determinations of medical futility are seldom so straightforward. Why is this so? Although situations vary, a common feature is that for most conditions, one can always do more to postpone death. Had doctors treated Betsy's second pneumonia with appropriate antibiotics, for example, she would not have awakened, but her pulmonary function would likely have recovered. Suppose she had left no advance directive. What would her doctors have recommended next? Because she was lying unresponsive in an acute care hospital with no likelihood of regaining consciousness but with other bodily functions more or less intact, they probably would have sought family approval to transfer her to another facility. California now contains more than thirty of them: freestanding chronic semi-ICUs for those with devastating neurological impairments. No patient walks or talks on the way in or ever regains consciousness, and none leaves alive. Some, though, remain residents for extended periods.

Is it "futile" to continue treating their infections and other metabolic derangements as they rather predictably arise? The problem with the futility concept, in my view, is that one may answer yes and another may respond no and both would be right, depending on where one set the physiological threshold. For Betsy's first neurologist, a patient moving a finger, even reflexively, was a sign of function that mandated aggressive care—"No one ever dies on my service, not if I can help it!" Much of the time he can get his way, for today's biomedical interventions can often sustain a person's basic metabolic functions for indefinite periods.

A patient who wants "everything done" or who has not indicated in advance that he or she wants otherwise may experience intensive interventions for an extended period before additional treatments are deemed futile. Moreover, if there is a legal dispute between an acute care team that believes futility has arrived and a patient's surrogate who demands more treatment, the courts almost always side with the surrogate. To give a sense of how Byzantine determinations of futility have become, as of 2007 a large hospital I know of is adopting an end-of-life policy that contains fifteen articles with many subclauses detailing how the residents and medical staff should address various aspects of futility. It was four years in the making and has become quite a bulky document. I wonder how the residents will manage to stuff it in their overflowing jacket pockets, let alone decipher it.

The problem with the new hospital policy, as with the concept of futility, is that the elephant in the room—dying—is seldom mentioned either on paper or in the day-to-day life of critical care decision making. Indeed, ICU doctors and patients' families can go for months without either ever mentioning the word. Dying is not what it was in 1950 or even 1970, as technology has transmuted the process from something that doctors and patients and their families could readily perceive into a range of contingent possibilities that often leave everyone in a quandary. Even so, would it not be wiser to recognize the elephant than to pretend it does not exist?

THE FRAGILE SELF: ELLEN'S ICU EXPERIENCE

What happens when the stakes are lower, when a seemingly reasonable ICU patient in the course of her illness insists on a plan of action that, although not wise, cannot be rejected by her physicians on the grounds that it is too dangerous? Can it be that assumptions behind the design and operation of ICUs cause them to function all too often as twilight zones in which "reason" and "autonomy" do not have their usual full meanings? In these situations, which are much more common than Betsy's, should physicians respect the intrinsic value of a person's autonomous decisions even as they wonder if that person may be making a mistake? Or should they assert an authority they used to rely on—"therapeutic privilege"—and restrain their patient's freedom?

Ellen, a professor of Italian, was running weekend marathons into her early forties. For reasons no one will ever understand, she awakened one morning in 2006 unable to catch her breath. Her husband called 911 and she was taken to an ER, where, over the next several hours, she went into respiratory failure. To preserve her life, the staff gave her sedatives and short-term paralytic agents so they could place a breathing tube in her windpipe (trachea) and thereby ventilate her mechanically. Her respiration stabilized and she was taken to the ICU. During the next few weeks, as she remained intubated, her kidneys and liver began to fail.

During this period she experienced awful physical distress on multiple levels. Though her body eventually recovered, in those weeks the inability of her liver and kidneys to perform their usual roles meant that part of her was poisoning the rest. That is how she felt, she said later—poisoned. Sick beyond sick, and certainly beyond caring about what had become the minor self-violations of pitiable moans and soiling herself, she longed just to sleep through it somehow. Despite regular sedation, however, she never slept soundly, and she felt she would never recover. Following day and night schedules of their own, ICU machines made their sounds, lights blinked on and off, and nurses and allied health personnel changed IVs and catheters and adjusted flow rates as doctors and medical students came and went and prodded and talked. To the extent she was aware, she valued their deft kindness like nothing else. When they were rude or inept, she felt her degradation was complete. She could not tell what time it was and there were no windows to the outside to cue her. She felt each moment of torment intensely, only to forget it the next. Whether the next moment was an hour or half a day away remained vague. Time seemed demolished. When she was by herself, she stared at the blank ceiling. In any case, she could do little. Not only did she feel too sick—too poisoned—to assert herself, but she could not even if she wished, at least not verbally, for she was being ventilated. (The larynx and trachea, exquisitely sensitive to foreign objects, never adapt easily to a breathing tube that chafes them. Just imagine how intensely you react if you feel yourself to be choking. Sedatives blunt the sensation, but patients report they still feel they are gagging and choking much of the time even when they are not. And then the intubated person must contend with the panic induced by temporarily having one's airway blocked while someone suctions its secretions.)

Ellen, who is not religious, nonetheless made endless deals with God to get the tube out. Dante's hell, whose inventive torments so fascinated her undergraduate students, lived in the form of the breathing tube in her airway. Indeed, what dominated her awareness in those weeks was not her sense of her body's sickness but rather her desire to "get this damned tube out!!"

Like many ICU patients, Ellen also experienced an even more searing sensation: the feeling that she was going in and out of "madness." Amplifying her loss of any reliable sense of who she was and what she was experiencing were her hallucinations. Ordinary interactions with the staff became frightening as reality and fantasy intermingled. She imagined, for example, that a staff member and some policemen were leaning over her, demanding that she file charges against a student bully who had been causing her real trouble before she became ill. On another occasion, a friend wearing a large crucifix around her neck loomed over her and asked if she wanted to see a priest. But how could this be, as Ellen was not Catholic and the friend was Jewish and lived abroad? Did the staff really have a drinking party in the middle of the ICU and make merry by ridiculing Ellen and the other patients? When her husband later told her that the ICU chaplain resembled her friend, she felt enormously relieved. She never did learn what to make of her delusion about the party.

Ellen experienced ICU psychosis or delirium—both terms are used—which occurs in a third or more of ICU patients and often leads to a post-traumatic stress disorder. Though she became weaned from the ventilator and began breathing on her own, her doctors wanted to leave the breathing tube in for a day or so in case she relapsed. Furious and determined to prevail, she countered with a clear written statement of her desire to be extubated. If her doctors would not oblige her, she let them know that she would take it out herself. Satisfied that she was mentally competent, they took out her breathing tube before they would have otherwise. After all, until she became sick she ran marathons, didn't she? When her breathing and other functions remained stable for another day, her doctors acceded to her new demand to go home even though they recommended a few more days in the hospital.

Ellen was thrilled to get home until she got there. Then she felt alarmingly and maddeningly fragile for many days. She could make little sense of what she had been through. "What was real?" she kept asking her husband about a particular memory. "What part was delusion?" Although her body recovered completely, she later said it took months to recover psychologically from her ICU experience. She continues to wonder whether she and the staff arranged the best outcome. Intellectual by nature and training, she wonders if an ethics of autonomy is really appropriate for someone as fragile as she was. What the ICU staff wonders about Ellen and others in her situation is the possibility of relapse after a patient initiates discharge. If that was to happen, or worse, how would the patient and her family and hospital staff—not to mention lawyers—have reviewed their decisions then?

The concept of autonomy, embraced initially as an ideal ethical mitten for almost all hands, may not work for the varied hands of patients in our hallucinogenic ICUs. Critical illness often drains one's reservoirs of personhood more deeply than any ICU replenishment, however vital, may refill. Indeed, desperate illnesses, the kind that involve multiple failing organs, often play the role of trickster for the afflicted and their caregivers alike. We physicians test for lucidity and mental competence by taking a series of snapshots, not a continuous film. When the patient's image in our single snapshot or small series of them looks adequate, as with Ellen, we assume the snapshots portray an underlying reality, particularly when the patient is telling us that they do.

If we express doubt, custom and law favor the patient's interpretation. Though physicians have the legal power in most jurisdictions to impose a seventy-two-hour hold on anyone whose behavior poses a grave threat to herself or the community, we are loath to exercise it upon someone who seems, as Ellen did, mentally normal. When a person remains fragile in ways that elude our snapshot tests, they and we can be fooled. Were we to petition a court for a restraint in these situations, which we hardly ever do, the courts almost always would side with the patient. The formal ethics of autonomy, based as they are on the assumption that a seemingly reasonable and willful patient has an intact psyche, have not been able to resolve this tension.

A very sick body's natural tendency to heal proceeds by fits and starts that easily mislead its psyche. In addition, the spaces, rhythms, and impersonal aggressiveness of ICU life compound the instability of self that so many patients experience. Putting aside for a moment Ellen's illness and medical regimen of ventilation, catheters, and possible interactions between her drugs—she received twelve different ones on most days—what is it about ICUs themselves that tends to drive patients crazy? What a bird flying overhead might notice provides a clue: the radial plan of most modern ICUs—individual cubicles arrayed around a central control station. Such a plan bears a striking resemblance to society's most explicitly controlling space, the modern maximum-security prison. Indeed, some American designers advertise their experience in devising both!

The model comes from Jeremy Bentham (1748–1832), the English polymath who argued for what he termed "utilitarian" approaches to philosophical and social issues. What Bentham particularly liked about his Panopticon, or "Inspection House," which he first proposed during the 1780s, was that its configuration of central all-seeing inspector and radial isolated cells served as an "engine" for "a new mode of obtaining power of mind over mind." Although Bentham was most concerned with prison reform, he drew explicit parallels between prison wardens and doctors, and between inmates and patients:

> *The whole prison would be perhaps a better hospital than any building known hitherto by that name . . . If any thing could still be wanting to show how far this plan is from any necessary connexion with severe and coercive measures, there cannot be a stronger consideration than that of the advantage with which it applies to hospitals . . . Here the physician and the apothecary might know with certainty that the prescription . . . had been administered at the exact time and in the exact manner in which it was ordered to be administered.*

Along with championing his Panopticon's ability to enforce surveillance and control, Bentham in other passages wrote with similar enthusiasm for its potential "economies" compared to extant alternatives: one prison inspector/nurse able to see and control many isolated prisoners/patients simultaneously.

If we wanted, we could go on at length about the incongruities of imagining maximum-security prisons and ICUs in the same expository breath. We might note that the Panopticon is not as good at accomplishing its goals—economical moral reform of prisoners and restoration of full health to patients—as Bentham claimed. It costs about the same to house a maximum-security young adult prisoner for a year as it does to send his law-abiding counterpart to Harvard, for example. And whatever else they are, ICUs are expensive to operate, with daily charges commonly running in the thousands of dollars. They, too, like prisons, have high recidivism rates, especially for the elderly with serious chronic diseases.

But it is their totalitarian dimensions that concern me most. Both maximum-security and ICU Panopticons insist not only that overwhelming power, surveillance, and control reside with the instruments of central authority, but also that the inmates/patients are to have none. When a sick person is experiencing life-threatening metabolic derangement, as in florid pulmonary edema, this makes medical sense. But that does not mean that control and surveillance need to be absolute moral imperatives governing all aspects of care for the very sick. Indeed, they are not the necessary *and* sufficient conditions for recovering personhood. The person, after all, still exists, and it is the person who will carry on—sick, well, or in between. It is the person inside the very sick body who needs all the help he or she can get. If this is so—and I will let Ellen stand as an example—then why do we design and operate most of our ICUs as if the person does not exist?

PLANETREE AND THE SPA

During the mid-1970s, Angie Theriot, then a young mother in San Francisco, began musing on the possibility of an alternative design after she spent time in a local hospital for a life-threatening condition. In her opinion, spending time in the ICU was more traumatic than enduring her acute illness, an impression reinforced by her experiences during the next year, when both her son and father-in-law underwent difficult hospitalizations. She was particularly troubled that she and her family spent so much time "in limbo," not knowing what was going on as doctors and staff hurried her or her relatives from one intervention to another. At a time when the Internet did not exist and medical libraries did not admit the public, she decided that patients needed their own sources of medical knowledge. In 1978 she founded a nonprofit organization, Planetree, which started as a medical library for the public—the Planetree Health Resource Center—next door to Presbyterian Hospital in San Francisco. In addition to being community-minded, warm, and extroverted, Theriot, whom I knew, was and is well connected—her husband, Richard, then published his family's newspaper, the *San Francisco Chronicle*. Within a short time, Planetree expanded its vision to include hospital spaces themselves. Thanks to local foundation support, the organization opened a thirteen-bed model medical-surgical facility at Presbyterian in 1985. Planetree, though still relatively small, has since gone nationwide, with a network of hospital model units and even an entire hospital following its principles.

Planetree's version of "putting the patient first" begins from the bedside out and encompasses everything a patient and his family might experience. Ironically, just as most extant ICUs follow an Enlightenment model—Bentham's Panopticon—Planetree's approach updates another Enlightenment health care model, the spa. Panopticon norms for color, lighting, and surface—generally white, harsh, and flat—give way to residential sensibilities: soothing color; a mix of lighting, some controlled by patients; and a variety of textures and patterns. Within reach and eyesight, patients can have personal memorabilia. They may wear their own pajamas, and visitors can sit in comfortable chairs near them; in some Planetree units they can sleep near them. Walls and sometimes ceilings display images of nature, typically realistic photographs or prints of trees and green or calm water. When possible, windows with patient-controlled coverings reveal pleasant outlooks. Adjacent visitor lounges have kitchenettes, healthy snacks, and small learning resource centers. The sounds of machines and hospital bustle are minimized. Massage therapists circulate regularly, musicians occasionally. Patients and their families are encouraged to be as knowledgeable as possible about their conditions and treatments. In hospital areas where Planetree has been introduced in a thorough way, surveys of patient *and* staff consistently report higher levels of satisfaction compared to standard counterparts. Although Planetree has not, to my knowledge, extended its approach into ICUs themselves, one can imagine how its ideas translate into those settings.

America has no lack of creative spa designers right now. Why not invite them into our ICUs? Facilitating a recovery of balance, which is the central purpose of the spa, is another way, albeit modest, of assisting a person to regain a sense of self. And should not recovery of self, to the degree that underlying disease permits, be the overall purpose for undergoing and delivering intense medical interventions? Power and control are only part of the picture, and to suggest otherwise is to pursue illusions that harm even as they try to help.

4

Elective Choices

Even if one has enjoyed general good health well into midlife, eventually one or another bodily organ, so quietly competent for decades, turns feckless. But when and how this happens varies considerably between individuals. The biological reality is that beginning in our mid-forties, we tend to age differently. If we were to look at changes in kidney function, for instance, we would find that up to our forties, most of us are alike in the rate and efficiency with which our kidneys clean our blood. After that, though, kidney functions begin to diverge. All one has to do to appreciate this in a visceral way is to attend one's twenty-fifth high school or college reunion and look around. Way back when we puzzled over the theorems of high school geometry, most of us looked to be more or less fifteen. A few decades later, however, some of us appear to be in our prime, or think we do, and others look and sound ready for retirement.

Sometimes our body's fecklessness expresses itself abruptly. On an icy winter sidewalk in Boston, Frank, who is sixty-two, slips, falls, and breaks his left hip. Assuming Frank's hip socket and thighbone are adequately calcified and not too arthritic, an orthopedic team will have him up and shoveling, or at least walking comfortably, in fairly short order. Sometimes the acute event is not a simple accident, but rather an expression of a serious underlying process. Suppose, for example, that Frank doesn't slip on that sidewalk but falls because he has experienced the sudden shock of a heart attack while shoveling snow. Fortunately for Frank, his wife, Mary, looking out the window, notices what has happened, calls 911, and paramedics come and take Frank to a nearby ER. Frank is admitted to the hospital, and the doctors, nurses, and techs tend to his emergent problems. Assuming the cause is straightforward—an otherwise good femoral neck that snaps from a fall, an acutely clogged coronary artery in a person without major coronary risk factors—Frank's experience of the illness will likely be straightforward. He'll be out of the hospital in a few days, actively convalescing, and soon able to return to his previous life only slightly the worse for wear. If Frank takes a little better care of himself after these events than he did before and enjoys some luck, then he may go on for another fifteen or twenty years before something else bad happens to his body.

Alternatively, suppose the events are the same—the inadvertent slip on the ice, the heart attack while shoveling snow—but their causes are more complicated and the benefit of their treatments is less straightforward. Whether it happens in our sixties or in our eighties, almost all of us will find ourselves enmeshed in complicated medical predicaments. We or our loved ones will have to make hard choices, and we will welcome none of them. Suppose, for example, that Frank and Mary are eighty-two and that their health has been declining for some time. They exist, they function, they may experience mostly good days and nights or parts of them. Nothing works as it used to, of course, as they say to themselves and their surviving friends and children, but it's not so bad. Still pretty good, in fact.

Many at this age still live independently, able to hear and see and read and drive. Others live with their children or in assisted living settings. When invited to talk about their lives, though, they let you know that even the tasks of daily living take immense willpower and care. Arthritis has made their joints fragile, which means that after Joe dies, Karen discovers that she cannot open a simple jar by herself anymore. So she stops buying food in jars, eats less, and doesn't tell her son. The elderly may not be sufficiently flexible to care for their feet (a chief focus of Hippocratic medicine, incidentally), which means they are more prone to falls, an important cause of significant disability. Diabetes may be slowly blinding them, an iffy heart valve finally conks out, a stroke makes speech or movement difficult, walking from the car to the market takes a cane and several long pauses for breath. "Now, what is my niece's name—Alice's daughter, her youngest. I *know* it, it's on the tip of my tongue . . . I can hardly do my errands without having to find a john to pee every forty-five minutes . . . Oh, damn it!"

And then something else bad happens. Whatever the proximate cause of the new insult, the underlying reality is that one's body's margin of safety has shrunk dramatically. In these situations, when some seemingly minor provocation pushes one or more of our organs over the precipice into a canyon of failure, what should we do? If we have private insurance or possess Medicare and/or Medicaid, most of us will see medical specialists who tend to specific failing parts, and they in turn will propose interventions. How do we choose among them when no choice will return us to what we were?

Before entering the realm of specialists and its seemingly endless offering of options, one might want to step back for a few moments and consider the demographics of life after eighty for almost anyone. What does "medical progress" mean for those of us in this age group? During the 1980s, a Swiss demographer, Arthur Imhof, published a series of papers that looked at human life and medical progress through the lens of four hundred years of life span records drawn from German archives. Even though his studies have received little mainstream attention, Imhof's findings may help frame the urgent choices that some of us face today. Among other things, what Imhof found about life expectancy after eighty is startling: it has barely changed in four hundred years!

If one were among the few who made it to age eighty in Berlin in 1600, for example, one could expect on average six more years of life. What I find astonishing is that Imhof also found that if one made it to age eighty in Berlin in 1980, one's average life expectancy was eighty-eight. Four hundred years of medical progress had gained the average octogenarian in Berlin—and by extension the rest of us who live in economically advanced societies—only about two more years of earthly life.

How can this be? Unlike our Renaissance forebears, we have specialist physicians with refined procedures for almost any bodily problem, not to mention dialysis machines, cardiac defibrillators, ventilators, ICUs, antibiotics, and hundreds of other drugs. And to what effect? Despite the ingenuity of medicine's panoply of late-life interventions, and putting aside their huge cost, inconvenience, and the suffering associated with using some of them, technologically advanced interventions appear to add little additional life for those in their ninth and tenth decades. To my knowledge, medical research has not yet determined why this is so.

The rub is that the comparatively few Berliners who made it to their mid-eighties in 1600 were allowed to die of "old age," which remained a common official cause of death until a few decades ago. Now that many make it into their ninth decade or more, nobody is allowed to officially die of old age, however. Instead, as Sherwin Nuland pointed out in his *How We Die* (1995), one is obliged to die of something specific, as old age is no longer an acceptable cause of death on a certificate. Instead, physicians must list a discrete diagnosis, such as pneumonia or kidney failure. But if a person reaches his late eighties or early nineties, is not dying from old age good enough?

If intense experience of specialist procedures and recurrent hospitalizations accomplish relatively little for those in their eighties, what approaches might help? Given biomedicine's cornucopia of choices, what are some pitfalls to avoid and routes to consider in navigating a prudent course?

TO WALK ON THE BEACH

Eliza and her late husband had enjoyed one of those extraordinary joint careers that combined creative work—they wrote screenplays together—with the uncluttered outdoor life that Southern California used to offer in abundance. He had died a decade ago, but Eliza, now in her mid-eighties, continued to spend her weekday mornings as she always had when he was alive—working on scripts in their beach house. Then she would go for a walk on the beach or along a canyon trail nearby, as she had with him. These routines continued until about two years ago, when her walks became shorter. Finally, she confined her activities to writing and running the necessary errands by car. It wasn't because she was weak that she stopped. Always strong, up to her early eighties Eliza still used her walking stick to whack the occasional rattler that threatened her or her corgis on their canyon strolls.

Eliza stopped walking simply because she had become too short of breath to venture along the beach or canyon paths. The reason, her internist soon determined, was that her heart's mitral valve, the one of its four that controls blood flow between the heart's small left chamber—the atrium—and large pumping chamber—the left ventricle—had given out. The result was that even minor exertion caused her, as it does others with similar conditions, to become easily short of breath. So her internist sent her to a cardiologist, and the cardiologist sent her to a cardiac surgeon. Confident she was a good operative candidate—Eliza was otherwise healthy—her surgeon recommended replacing her mitral valve. She was optimistic that with the new heart valve, Eliza's breathing would improve and she would regain the stamina she had lost when her original valve failed.

In a narrow sense, all her doctors' predictions for their intervention proved true. Eliza underwent the valve replacement and could walk farther and more easily than she had been able to in years. But within a few months she was not sure her new valve had made her life better. Though her breathing was no longer much of an issue, something else had come up that impinged on her ability to function. Indeed, Eliza barely left her house anymore, for she had become afraid to drive. She began calling her son in a distant city ten times a day to complain about her memory—it was gone. So gone, her son later said to me, that she could not remember how often she called him. No wonder she did not want to venture out: she could not remember her way home. Eliza knew this was happening—senility—and her accelerating memory loss often pushed her into despair. Fortunately, she and her son, an only child, were close, and she and her late husband had accumulated some money. Upon her request, Eliza's son, who is a college friend of mine, arranged private care for his mother in the home she loved and flew in weekly to spend time with her. Even so, Eliza died within two years of her mitral valve replacement.

During those two years, Eliza told her son more than once that if she had her late life to do over, she would rather have gone with an oxygen bottle and short walks and kept her mind than have the new valve and quickly decline into what she called "gaga land." Until the surgery, Eliza's memory had always been acute. What her son wanted to know from me when we met a few months after her death was whether his mother's mitral valve operation provoked her memory loss. No longer the laid-back surfer I knew in our youth, my friend had become an intense venture capitalist in Silicon Valley, and he wanted an explanation. At first, not wanting his anger at her death to derail his grief, I demurred. As we both knew, I said, I was no heart expert. "I know that," he responded. "I'm talking to heart experts." What they told him, he related, confirmed in greater detail what I have read and gleaned from my ER work: a significant percentage of elderly people who go on cardiac bypass pumps for more than a short time subsequently experience substantial loss of mental function. We were walking through a redwood grove as we talked, and I was thinking of the trees and their high green light as I listened to the rage in my friend's voice. He wanted to sue his mother's cardiac surgeon and her hospital, both of which have excellent reputations. What he really wanted from me, I thought, was not my knowledge of heart surgery, which we both knew was (and is) slender, but the confirmation one longtime friend can give another for some important decision. "Why didn't they tell us that!" my friend repeated with feeling. "Why didn't they give us the full picture? Surgeons aren't supposed to be salesmen, right? If that surgeon knew there was a 20 or 30 percent chance my mother would lose her memory, shouldn't she have told us that? Isn't that negligence?"

When we talked by phone a few weeks later and my friend was calmer, I mentioned that the development of almost every invasive procedure, whether surgical or medical, follows a learning curve of accumulating knowledge. Animal models, which provide the usual experimental substrate for human interventions, rarely correlate tightly with initial attempts on humans. Successes, failures, and complications in the early human procedures lead to refinements that tend to improve outcomes. But it takes a number of procedures and a significant follow-up period, sometimes a large number and a longish follow-up, to make the value of a refinement visible. Ditto for the perception of a significant risk or long-term complication. And even then, one often remains in the dark. Several factors account for the murkiness, especially among the very old.

"Let's put this in the context of your mother," I said to my friend. Prior to the early 1990s, not many U.S. cardiac surgeons did open heart surgery on people in their mid-eighties and early nineties. Without having the data to know just what the risks might be, they nonetheless assumed the risks were not worth the benefits, so they did not recommend the interventions. This is still the case outside the United States. Few chronically ill octogenarians and nonagenarians elsewhere in the world elect to undergo major invasive procedures on *any* of their body's major organs. Their physicians tend not to recommend them, their very old patients tend not to demand them, and their health care systems usually will not pay for them. But in the United States, the reverse holds true for each of these steps, especially when it comes to surgery on the very elderly with failing hearts and advanced solid cancers. Replacing the heart valve of a ninety-year-old, if not exactly commonplace, is no longer rare in America. Putting aside for the moment the question of why this is so, the scientific reality is that physicians and medical science do not know very much about the physiological effects of major heart surgery on eighty- and ninety-year-old bodies. Most of the knowledge of how these operations work in humans is based on younger populations, and good animal models for major surgery on senescent hearts simply don't exist. The general lack of knowledge pertains to major interventions on other organ systems in the very elderly as well.

"So what's your point?" my friend interjected. "I've got a lawyer who thinks we have a good case. Failure to adequately disclose risks, therefore lack of informed consent, therefore breach of fiduciary duty, therefore gross negligence—almost open-and-shut, she says . . . I called to get your thoughts, not an article abstract."

I did not like my friend's testiness or his pursuit of vengeance. "What I've been saying," I responded, "is that knowledge of risks in major heart surgery on the very elderly, like risk profiles in anything else, requires data. *Now* we know what we didn't a few years ago about putting eighty-five-year-olds on bypass pumps—if they're on for very long, a significant percentage lose short-term memory and other cognitive function.

"So if you want to sue for damages based on your mother's surgeon's negligence for not disclosing risk," I continued, "you and your lawyer should look closely at the disclosure section on the consent forms she signed. I'll wager the forms said something about potential damage to the brain and central nervous system. They may even have said that bypass pumps in the very elderly carry significant risks to mental function. Either way, I think your mother's surgeon has a reasonable defense. Your mother was proud of negotiating on her own with the studios, right? And you were there with her in the surgeon's office, and you make your living doing investment deals. When it comes to the fine print of contracts and disclosure, you can hardly claim you two were naive babes in the woods. Whether the surgeon should have spent more time with your mother before she recommended the surgery is something else. [My friend said she spent eight minutes.] But my hunch is, you won't prevail."

Neither of us brought up the issue again, but when I saw my friend next—we usually get together in California during summers—his wife told me they had decided not to sue.

"CORNUCOPIA OF CHOICES" OR THICKET?

Earlier I used the phrase *biomedicine's cornucopia of choices.* As we specialist doctors, hospital administrators, and biomedical corporation executives see ourselves in relation to the world, *cornucopia* and *choices* seem apt, for we like to think of ourselves as purveyors of abundant feasts of marvelous and life-affirming possibilities.

The words suggest to our patients that the array of choices is rather like some splendid buffet line, a medical version of Thanksgiving dinner at the Ritz. But for many in late life with serious chronic problems, the rhetoric of elective choices ends up ringing hollow, as it did for Eliza. When faced with a range of "treatment options" for a serious chronic problem, many elderly patients have told me they find themselves not strolling in a consumerist paradise, but wandering endlessly through a thicket. Why is this so?

Although each ill person's situation is truly unique, there are general factors that make notions of "elective choices" problematic. They tend to operate under the surface for patients and doctors alike. This section briefly describes a threefold scheme a number of researchers in diverse fields have found to be useful in elucidating the murk. My premise is that knowing this scheme and how it operates may help one navigate the maze of late-life medical choices.

Along with the striking images of our country taken on high from satellite cameras, another remarkable series of images of today's America consists of maps of how medical resources are used in different parts of the United States. Known as the Dartmouth Atlas of Health Care, these regularly updated maps, which one can easily find at their website—www.dartmouthatlas.org—or on Google, are the visual representations of a long-term study of outcomes in American health care. Using epidemiology, economics, and statistics, the Dartmouth group's graphics reveal several truths that are almost impossible for any individual patient or physician to notice. The most striking, which I alluded to earlier in noting Imhof's review of four hundred years of German life span data, is that for those in their mid-seventies or beyond, *more is not better*, especially when it comes to the seemingly endless rounds of specialist visits and aggressive treatments common in late-life medical care.

It seems counterintuitive, I know, but the Dartmouth analyses, which adjust comparisons to account for demographic variables such as average age in a population, have been accumulating for more than a decade and are considered persuasive by many in the social sciences. As Eliza's story suggests, analyses by the Dartmouth group and others confirm that open heart cardiac surgery accomplishes little for those with heart failure in their late eighties, just as renal dialysis for those with chronic renal failure does little to extend the amount or quality of life for those in that age group. Meanwhile, some modest interventions, often overlooked, may matter a lot.

When one looks at the Dartmouth Atlas's image of Boca Raton, Florida, for example, what one sees is not the low-lying retirement enclave for the affluent depicted in conventional maps and photographs, but instead a virtual Everest of medical specialists and doctor visits and procedures and hospitalizations. In comparison, Dartmouth Atlas depictions of High Plains states like the Dakotas don't look high at all but rather like valleys with plenty of generalist physicians but many fewer specialists, operations, and hospital beds per capita. To the degree that concepts like "quality-adjusted life year" can measure an individual's health experience, it is not in Boca Raton that an elderly person will live longer. Southeast Florida may have that great winter climate and contain beehives of competent specialist physicians and high-tech facilities, but if one is sixty-five or older, one will do better on average making sure one's vehicle's engine doesn't freeze up overnight in Pierre in

February than rubbing SPF-30 sunscreen on one's shoulders by a pool in South Florida—at least in terms of long-term health. And that person—or Medicare—will save a lot of money besides.

PREFERENCES: YOUR "CHOICES" ARE
SELDOM REALLY YOURS

If, strange as it seems, *more is not better*, how should one go about making individual choices? The first thing to realize—and it is also counterintuitive—is that an individual's preference for one approach over another is not as *individual* as one might think. When it comes to discretionary surgery—Eliza's choice of a mitral valve replacement and the bypass pump in preference to medical management of her shortness of breath—it is the practice style of the doctors in the community that really counts. More than the particulars of a disease or environmental factors, what happens to patients depends on what the local specialists are used to doing.

The importance of a community's prevailing medical opinion first became apparent over seventy years ago. During the 1930s, British pediatrician J. Alison Glover became intrigued with variations in tonsillectomy rates among British schoolchildren. How can it be, he wondered, that a child in one district is ten times as likely to have his or her tonsils out compared to a child in another? It could not have been a variance in commonplace childhood throat infections, as their incidence varied little from district to district. As Glover sought to explain the variation, he was able to use his data to rule out many illness-related and environmental factors. But the clincher came when a new district health officer happened to take over one of the school groups Glover had been following. Within a year of the new officer's arrival, tonsillectomy rates in his district fell by a factor of ten, a decline Glover attributed to a change in "medical opinion."

How might one translate a 1930s insight about treatments for British youngsters with inflamed tonsils into wisdom for older Americans today? Suppose you are elderly and have a chronic problem with your hip, knee, or back—the kind of problem for which one commonly consults an orthopedist. You might think, based on Glover's findings, that if you live where there are many orthopedists trained to do surgery, you will be offered mostly surgical treatments compared to non-surgical treatments. That is true—the greater the density of procedure-oriented providers in an area, the greater the number of procedures that get performed there—but only up to a point. Since Glover's day, and especially in America, not only have specialties proliferated, but almost every specialty has divided into subspecialties. All orthopedists are alike in the sense that all cardiologists and all neurosurgeons are also alike—members of each group have experienced a lengthy common training in their particular organ system. But after that, each specialist tends to subspecialize so that he or she repeatedly performs only a small number of the specialty's repertoire of possible treatments. In short, each proceduralist develops a procedural "signature."

According to Dartmouth Atlas data, what determines the particular treatments offered to any single patient depends not so much on the patient's preferences or the density of specialists in their area, but instead on the subspecialty "signatures" of those experts. Also, specialists with similar "signatures" tend to congregate. For patients with similar presentations, orthopedists in Fort Myers, which is on Florida's mid–Gulf Coast, for example, perform knee, hip, and back surgeries at twice the rate of their Miami counterparts to the southeast.

In short, physicians, like almost every other kind of professional, do what they are trained to do. And given that most specialists train for increasingly longer periods in the mastery of what becomes a small number of interventions—Stanford neurosurgery residents now train for seven years beyond medical school, for instance, and many do fellowships for a year or two after that—it behooves one to know how the specialist tends to approach a particular problem. For those with a rare or even unusual condition it may make sense to use one's medical contacts and the Internet to find the one or two or six subspecialists who have devoted their careers to their problem, as they are likely conversant with the most promising treatments. But if your particular problem is more common—poignant but relatively routine, like Eliza's increasing shortness of breath in her mid-eighties—it may be equally crucial to get a good sense of your specialist's practice preferences—his or her thought style or "signature"—before signing on for an intervention. This may not be easy. The specialist you see may have a tendency to present his or her approach to your situation as *the* approach. If so, he or she may be reticent or show impatience with your questions. When my ER colleague Mike first learned he had cancer, for example, he went to a couple of different surgeons before he found one that he could work with. Mike was medically savvy and not intimidated by the settings in which medical consultations take place. Most of us do not have his personality or training. But his questions were important and reasonable. Most specialists will make sure they know plenty about any patient's body, or at least the organ system or disease process that falls within their purview. You need, however, to let them know about the person inside your body. What has your illness experience been for you, and what matters to you going forward? For example: how important is mental agility to you when weighed against other functions, such as exercise stamina? Had Eliza's doctor been able to figure out the answer, her life might have gone differently. I continue to be astonished (and saddened) at how little time our patients take with us and we with them before making important decisions. Eliza's son said that her surgeon spent eight minutes with them before they "decided" on her mitral valve replacement. Eight minutes of actual "face time" is not uncommon for such consultations, so studies report. That we physicians settle for such limited conversations makes a mockery of the shared decision making that stands behind true elective choice. Careful listening has such important consequences that to do otherwise may lead to what none of us, doctors and patients alike, wants: an outcome, like Eliza's, in which the doctor performs a "success" that the patient experiences as a failure.

Fortunately, recent development of patient-oriented decision aids may help one navigate among the various treatment options for some chronic problems. When available, they have proven to be immensely helpful. During the 1990s, for example, two large HMOs gave their men diagnosed with enlarged prostates a straight-forward analysis that compared the results of "watchful waiting" with surgery (prostatectomy). Follow-up showed that those who received the guide elected surgery at a rate 40 percent less than those in a control group whose members did not receive the analysis, yet they experienced similar or better outcomes. Other studies have confirmed the general observation that truly informed patients with chronic problems who are offered a choice between conservative or invasive approaches tend to prefer the former.

Women with early-stage breast cancer now may find excellent guides on the Internet or in a bookstore that compare lumpectomy with mastectomy for similar tumors. Thus informed, these women and their doctors can make truly shared decisions about treatment. People experiencing chest pain due to coronary artery disease may likewise find good information about medical management versus surgery for their heart problem.

But for those in late life, few decision aids exist. The analyses are only as good as the comparative data that stand behind them. A large number of midlife women have experienced early breast cancer, and therefore researchers can make statistically valid comparisons between different treatment approaches. But the number of eighty-five-year-olds with any particular problem is comparatively small. The same applies to infants in similar situations: sufficient evidence rarely exists concerning the risks, benefits, and uncertainties that their parents need to make valid comparisons. At either end of the life spectrum, it is the idiosyncratic practice styles of local specialists—*their* preferences, not the patients'—that determine the menu of choices.

SETTINGS: IF YOU BUILD IT, THEY WILL COME

If treatment choices often turn out to be other than one's own, the number of late-life doctor visits and the amount of time one passes in hospitals may also be determined by others. This is especially true for those suffering from serious chronic illnesses such as heart failure, chronic lung disease, and cancer. Although a specialist's procedural preferences may have a lot to do with what choices patients are offered, how often patients see their specialists and the frequency and length of late-life hospitalizations have little to do with conscious choices of the specialists or their patients. The statement deserves repeating because it runs so counter to either's sense of agency. What may not be apparent to patients *or* doctors is the role that settings—densities of hospital beds in a given area and numbers of available visits to an area's specialists—play in the scope of medical practice. It is these two seemingly humdrum facts, not individual patient or physician preference, that shape the frequency and extent of late-life medical encounters.

In the 1989 movie *Field of Dreams*, Ray Kinsella, the farmer played by Kevin Costner, hears a ghostly voice say, "If you build it, he will come." Eventually, Kinsella builds "it"—a regulation baseball diamond—in his cornfield, and "he"—the ghost of Shoeless Joe Jackson and those of his White Sox teammates from the 1919 World Series—shows up to play. Much the same can be said for hospital beds, especially for the medical (nonsurgical) conditions we commonly experience in late life. Beginning in the early 1960s, a researcher named Milton Roemer became intrigued with how Americans use our hospitals. What Roemer's studies kept demonstrating is that hospital beds, once built, will be used, no matter how many there are. Subsequent researchers have dubbed this relationship between the supply of hospital beds per capita and their utilization "Roemer's law" in his honor.

Boston and New Haven, for example, are not far apart, and both have excellent hospitals and medical training programs. One would think that an elderly sick Bostonian would be as likely to be hospitalized as his Connecticut counterpart afflicted with the same kind of problem. At least that's what doctors who have practiced in both places thought—we do things about the same here and there. But if one looks at the ill Bostonians as a group, they are 60 percent more likely to be hospitalized for a given medical condition than if they lived in New Haven. The determining factor, according to the studies, is that Boston has a much higher number of hospital beds per capita than New Haven. As in *Field of Dreams*, if you build it, they will come. (The above correlation does not hold for those who urgently need major surgery. Frank broke his hip in Boston, but if he had broken it in Missoula or St. Louis he would be as likely, on average, to be hospitalized and treated much as if he were in Boston.)

When it comes to the end of life—someone's last six months—the regional variation in the amount of time the average person spends in a hospital bed becomes striking. If a person's life is winding down from chronic illness in Manhattan, which has the highest rate of late-life hospitalization in the country, he will likely spend around twenty days in hospital. In comparison, in the region with the lowest rate, he would spend six. As far as I know, Mike was not aware of the particular hospital bed situation in our part of the country. All he knew as he experienced the terminal stage of his cancer was that he wanted to spend his final months as comfortably as possible in his home. In order to do that, he and his wife Marge focused their efforts on securing excellent palliative care through in-home hospice nurses.

For their part, hospitals, especially those connected with medical schools, compete routinely to be labeled among the "best," as in the annual list of "best hospitals in the United States" that *U.S. News and World Report* publishes. Since most of us usually stick with one group of doctors and one hospital during late-life illnesses, we may want to choose one of these "best" facilities for our care. In her final months, Eliza returned several times for hospitalization to a top hospital in Los Angeles. She happened to spend more than three weeks of her final six months there, including several days in its ICUs. Had Eliza received her care in San Francisco, where her son lived, and gone into Moffitt Hospital at the University of California—also widely considered among the "best"—she likely would have been in hospital only a little more than a week and not admitted to an ICU.

Compilers of lists of "best hospitals" look at many variables, but to my knowledge they do not include rates of late-life hospitalization among them. Yet it is the custom of particular hospitals—and I am speaking of the "best" ones—not a patient's particular illness, that determines how often one is likely to be in hospital and how aggressively one will be treated while there. Even among top hospitals in the same university system, such as UCLA and UCSF, significant variations exist for end-of-life care. According to one good study, patients loyal to UCLA spend over three times more days in its ICUs during their final six months than their counterparts at UCSF do in its. Yet no evidence exists that patients do better at UCLA.

Similar relationships prevail concerning numbers of available office appointments for most subspecialties: if the appointment slots exist, they get filled.

Elliott Fisher's group at Dartmouth and other studies of end-of-life care at our "best" medical centers confirm my own experiences practicing medicine in some of them: *more usually means less*. Specifically, sick elderly people who endure the aggressive treatments that our "best" medical centers routinely administer near the end of their lives tend not to survive any longer than those who avoid such treatments. All that has progressed, in most of these situations, is the length and agony of dying. In 1600 the few eighty-six-year-olds around died short deaths, usually from infections; four hundred years later our octogenarians tend to live a couple of years longer, but they—we—have traded the abrupt departures of our elderly forebears for a new kind of oblivion: the drawn-out and agonizing dying that occurs routinely, especially (and paradoxically) in our "best" places.

"Medical progress" is real for many diseases during much of their course. Prior to the discovery of insulin in the 1920s, for example, a child with diabetes could expect to live but a few years; now that child can look forward to an almost normal life span, albeit one replete with intense medical management. Even so, "medical progress" doesn't mean much at the end. When it comes to elective choices for managing late-life chronic illness, I need to acknowledge the paucity of research in this area. Although hundreds of billions of dollars are spent every year in this country on medical care for people in the last six months of life, only a few million support the kind of research the Dartmouth Atlas group has undertaken.

Another frustrating reality is that unlike terminal cancers, which tend to have predictable final paths, the diseases that kill the majority of the very old tend not to follow predictable courses. Suppose, for example, that a woman has diabetes and hypertension and some heart, kidney, and lung disease—a common late-life picture. She experiences a collapse of some sort and is brought to an ER or ICU. Unless that person is truly at the end—little or no blood pressure, lungs so stiff that mechanical ventilation is problematic, signs of minimal brain stem function—we doctors cannot accurately predict how long she will last or what degree of function she might regain. Yet her prospects for five-year survival may differ little from someone with Stage IV lung cancer.

Consequently, critical care physicians start to do things, and for a short time they often prop up the patient's kidney function, blood oxygen, and so forth. We know the person is sinking, but when her family asks "How long?" or the equivalent, we cannot tell them. Or, if we make a prediction, we are often wrong. Is the person before us dying? Should we be thinking about hospice care? The families ask us these questions and we ask them of each other. At these times, we, they, and the patient are in the thicket, and none of us can see more than a few feet ahead. Unless the patient or her family speaks clearly and decisively about what they want, and sometimes even when they do, we doctors either dither or just muddle on.

In hindsight—the Dartmouth Atlas specialty—it is easy to see that our care has been futile, at least as measured across a population. Its futility, though sensed, is not as apparent at the individual sick person's bedside in real time. Because most physicians and the medical science on which we depend are myopic in these moments, and because provider opinions and hospital customs determine one's choices more commonly than perceived, I have been emphasizing the value of taking a long view—call it the Imhof version—of late life. It will not assuage any specific problem, but it does provide a perspective to appreciate the shape of late-life critical illness and the amount of intense specialist attention one might decide to endure as life winds down.

The constraints on choices, notions of medical futility, and a general insistence on doing "everything possible" near the end all speak to the radical transformation of the meanings of *life*, *death*, and *salvation* that has occurred during the past four hundred years in the West. In 1600 the Catholic peasants whose life span records Imhof studied shared a cultural outlook in which some version of a believer's life stretched to eternity. They and their early Protestant counterparts alike believed that earthly life was both individual and communal, and in any case, thanks to their faith, divine mercy, and the Holy Spirit, it was only a stepping-stone to an eternal life. Now, even if we are fundamentalist Christians, most of us behave medically as if our earthly life in our particular body is all we have. We in the West, and in America especially, have persuaded ourselves that one's individual *materiality* is a better deal than their notions of one's *spirit*. Perhaps it is; I venture that most of us hope so, anyway. This hope, in my view, is the deep reason that motivates doctors and patients alike to operate up to a patient's earthly end as if *more is better* even though most studies, as well as my own and others' bedside experiences, suggest the wisdom of gentler and more humble approaches.

EFFECTIVE CARE, OR THE IMPORTANCE OF MINDING THE DETAILS

If reliance on intense specialism and technology do not accomplish much and in fact may harm, what can those of us with serious chronic problems do to help ourselves? If God and genius lie in attention to details, the good news is that for common chronic problems—heart disease, breast cancer, diabetes, and the like—the little things often count for a lot. One pill of baby aspirin, for example, costs a penny or two. Yet giving that aspirin pill promptly to someone experiencing a heart attack improves his or her chances for a good outcome almost as much as anything else physicians do emergently. If one wants to reduce the incidence of advanced breast cancer, ditto for the benefits of mammograms every two years for women aged fifty-two to sixty-nine. So, too, for the benefits to diabetics of regularly monitoring their hemoglobin (HbA1c), undergoing annual eye exams, and taking meticulous care of their feet.

Mammograms and hemoglobin monitoring cost more than an aspirin pill, but they do not cost much compared to a round of chemotherapy or an hour in an ICU, and they may succeed in keeping one from experiencing either. Each of them is an example of what researchers in health care outcomes—the Dartmouth Atlas folks and their colleagues elsewhere—call "effective care." Based on large-scale studies of outcomes or evidence of randomized clinical trials, *effective care* consists of therapeutic interventions—the pill of baby aspirin when someone hits the ER with severe chest pain—and diagnostic tests—the mammogram every two years for women in their fifties or sixties—whose benefits so outweigh the risks that almost all patients in those specific categories should receive them.

Taken as a whole, the interventions of effective care form the substrate of what researchers call "best-practice guidelines" and "evidence-based medicine." While these recommendations are useful for the common problems—such as asthma, breast cancer, heart attacks, and diabetes—that afflict millions, the statistical concepts that inform them do not have much relevance for rare conditions. Putting rare conditions aside, then, how does one avail oneself of the benefits of these practice guidelines and their effective care?

Subscribers to a comprehensive prepaid group like Kaiser Permanente or Group Health (Seattle) that operates its own system of providers and facilities tend to be treated according to such guidelines, as these groups have the records, data, and commitment to evaluate what works and what does not. In turn, they can inform their practitioners and patients about them. The informational guide for men diagnosed with enlarged prostates is one example of this; another is that most Kaiser patients with diabetes do get tested regularly for the HbA1c, and their midlife women get mammograms every two years.

Those who are covered through Medicare but who do not belong to a Kaiser-like group plan and, instead, find doctors as they need them may or may not be getting the benefits of best-practice guidelines. Beth McGlynn, a health quality researcher, and her colleagues published a study in *The New England Journal of Medicine* in 2003 that analyzed data on 439 different quality measures for different conditions affecting large numbers of patients. What they found, discouragingly, was that patients received recommended care only a little more than half the time—about 55 percent.

Unfortunately, just possessing a Medicare or Medicaid card (or substantial private insurance) does not assure one of being among the 55 percent. Other factors come into play. One reason is that Medicare and Medicaid, and Aetna for that matter, are huge bureaucracies. They are so of necessity, but they have not configured their infrastructure, as prepaid plans like Kaiser have, to encourage widespread adoption of best-practice guidelines. Instead, they reimburse individual providers or groups of providers and individual hospitals for treatment on what amounts to a fee-for-service basis.

Many Medicare patients have told me and others that they wonder "Who's in charge?" Especially in areas replete with specialists, like Boca Raton or almost any affluent suburban enclave, patients may be getting lots of medical attention from a variety of experts, but experience little or no *coordinated* care. Where lack of coordination reigns, adherence to best-practice guidelines tends to languish. Most organ-based specialists—cardiologists, neurologists, nephrologists and the like—are expert in their one area. One consequence is that if a person just sees different specialists for different problems, none of these physicians, however well-meaning, is likely to have the big picture. Routine maintenance—the details of effective care—may fall through the cracks.

Indeed, a Dartmouth study of "effective care" in 2004 revealed that patients in areas with a high concentration of specialists and high Medicare spending receive less high-quality effective care than patients who live in areas with lower Medicare spending but a greater density of general practitioners. Primary care physicians—the GPs, family medicine doctors, and general internists of the medical world—are trained broadly, and increasingly, to serve patients as their coordinators of care along best-practice lines. In effect, they incorporate into their individual or group practices a wide-ranging awareness of what will likely work best for their patients' common problems. In other words, to be among the 55 percent receiving "effective care" for common chronic problems, one's best tactic is to work with a generalist physician or within a comprehensive prepaid plan like Kaiser. Within either framework—the small generalist practice or the large prepaid plan—one has a better chance of making truly informed choices than by shopping on one's own among the medical specialist boutiques. Regular attention toward you as a person from a good primary care physician and vigilance toward all your problems likely will accomplish more than ad hoc consultations with specialists, no matter how technically refined they may be.

5

Reflections on the Plight of Sick Children

On March 8, 2006, *The New York Times* published a front-page color photo of an emaciated African boy holding his hands in front of his eyes. The boy was black, and at first I assumed the photo accompanied a story about refugees from the ongoing genocide in Darfur. But I was mistaken. The caption stated the boy had AIDS and was seven years old. The media have published many similar images during recent years, and they continue to stop the heart. This one jolted me for an additional reason: the *Times* revealed the child's name. AIDS carries a huge familial stigma in the United States, and an even larger one elsewhere. Was the boy, who appeared close to death, not entitled to some shred of respect, including his privacy? Suppose he had been white and lived in Grosse Pointe or Greenwich—would the *Times* photographer have even gotten within camera distance? (If the boy had been an American, incidentally, publication of his name, photograph, and AIDS diagnosis would have violated federal statutes that carry criminal penalties. Also, if he had been in America, the boy might be infected with HIV, but these days he would be unlikely to have AIDS, for he would have been receiving treatments that inhibit HIV's replication.)

Publication by the *Times* of the boy's diagnosis along with his face and name illustrates a general confusion our society manifests toward children and their moral space, especially when it comes to medical issues. Among other questions, what boundaries should we observe around sick children? Along with a moral claim on our resources, does a child not have some irreducible claim to the dignity of his or her own person? If so, what might such a claim mean for his or her parents? What roles should doctors, hospitals, the legal system, and the media play when the medical stakes for a child are high? It is difficult to have answers to these questions for children and their parents, and in some respects single answers probably do not exist.

Yet matters have become urgent. Several developments, some of them not readily apparent, have shifted the ground rules and upped the ante during recent decades, and not just for children, as what affects them in dramatic ways routinely occurs more quietly in adults. Current practices do not provide as much guidance or support as one might like.

BRITNEY, 2005

The poignancy of the boy's expression in the *Times* photograph calls forth memories of another very ill seven-year-old I met recently. In terms of medical resources, their situations do not compare, for she received not too little treatment, but rather, too much. What they share, ironically, is that adults involved with each of them did not respect the child as a person in his and her own right. I shall call the girl Britney, and her situation starkly illustrates a truism that anyone who works with children learns early on: in general, one can only do as well with a sick child as one can with her parents. A medical relationship with a child is not the simple dyad of doctor and patient, as it usually is with adults, but instead a three- or four-sided relationship in which the child, the parents, occasional others, and we doctors and nurses all play roles. None of this is new—other than for extraordinary lapses, most American parents have determined their children's care since the nation began. But the new aggressiveness of our treatments has complicated the picture.

In theory, anyone involved with a hospital patient—the patient, her doctors and nurses, her family, a hospital administrator—may request a consultation with the hospital's ethics committee. Those who request them tend to want advice on the "best possible outcome." Most of the time, doctors are the ones making the requests, which is what happened with Britney. In her situation, though, any of the adults involved—her mother and father, her nurses, her physicians, an administrator—might have called us, for all were at their wits' end. It took but a glance at Britney to undertand why. Britney had spent almost three of her seven years coping with one of the rarest and most devastating forms of solid cancer in children. Perhaps because it started quietly in her nascent genitalia, a few months passed before she or her parents suspected Britney's occasional "cramps down there" might be a sign of something "really wrong." They lived outside a small town, and although her local physician promptly arranged for them a consultation with a pediatric cancer specialist in a nearby large city, the cancer had already spread—metastasized—to her surrounding body. Given the aggressiveness of Britney's cancer cell type and the extent of its early spread, none of her cancer center's physicians entertained hope of a substantial remission or cure for her. Alas—at least in hindsight—they did not tell her parents that. Instead, according to her mother, they said little about her chances and used a word—*temporize*—that may sound more benign to lay ears than to professional ones. Of course, the family wanted all the temporizing measures available, and who can blame them? As the cancer spread, therefore, Britney experienced, along with several rounds of chemotherapy and radiation, the amputation of her legs, hips, and finally, her lower pelvis. These interventions occurred over almost three years. Along the way, one or another Gulf Coast physician or cancer treatment group tried to persuade Britney's parents to hold off. The treatments were no longer therapies, they said, but simply mutilations. They would not help Britney achieve a period of remission, but instead would only prolong her agony.

Her parents, however, did not agree. For her mother especially, Britney's fate lay in the hands of God. Britney's mother was a born-again Christian, and she *knew* God wanted Britney's doctors to do *everything*. She and her pastor both expressed faith that a miracle would happen. Britney's father was not so sure, but then he did not feel as "born-again" as her mother. In fact, he drank and used drugs and was in and out of the family home. Hospital records noted that he visited his daughter occasionally, though not with the regularity of her mother, and that once he agreed with medical recommendations for "comfort care." But during group meetings with his wife and Britney's cancer team, he was no match for the girl's mother.

The records contain no trace of Britney's voice.

Twice the records indicate that physicians in different hospitals refused to go along with the mother's demands. On those occasions, Britney's mother, after shouting at the doctors, took her daughter home against medical advice. When Britney experienced her next crisis, her mother would go to a different large city and its ER, then lobby for aggressive care once Britney was admitted and the crisis abated.

By the time we saw Britney, she appeared utterly exhausted. What remained of her—her upper body—appeared even more grotesque than it would have otherwise because a tumor oozing blood extruded from what was left of her vagina. With her longest bones amputated, her remaining bone marrow, the area in the body that produces most of the blood's components, could no longer keep up, which is why she had commenced bleeding. For a day or two, transfusions could bolster her blood and stop the bleeding before their effects dissipated. This could not go on, for her blood type was so rare and her need so great that continuing her transfusions would soon deplete the Gulf Coast region's reserves of her type. Her doctors asked us to consider her situation because they did not want to exhaust a rare and important medical resource for a futile purpose.

One may ask, Why did her doctors let things go so far? Why did they not stand up to the mother sooner? Certainly, some of her physicians tried, but her mother went right around them and arranged other care in different cities. Even so, was there no way to prevent such a futile and cruel undertaking? Theoretically, the legal system provides a method. During the late 1980s and the 1990s, when wise use of scarce medical resources emerged as an important issue, physicians and ethicists, along with hospitals and their attorneys, went to the courts several times to gain court orders to halt treatments they argued were "futile." Even when doctors can agree that more care would be futile, legal definitions of futility remain imprecise. The decisions of several courts suggest that futility, like beauty, lies in the eyes of the beholder. Repeatedly, judges have expressed reluctance to override parents' petitions for continued treatments for their terminally ill children, regardless of physicians' testimony that such treatments were futile. Nonetheless, with Britney we were prepared to go to court to halt the transfusions. According to the lawyers, we had a reasonably solid case, not on the grounds of futility per se but instead on utilitarian grounds: the unfairness to the public of jeopardizing an important regional resource for the dubious benefit of a single person.

Like many hospital ethics committees, ours followed a process where a small subcommittee—in our case two—would visit with the family and patient and report back to the larger group. My colleague and I very much wanted some time alone with Britney, but this proved difficult. Her mother was more or less camping in Britney's room, and she would not let us near her without also being present. Indeed, the bedside had become crowded, for not only was Britney's mother almost always there, but also her pastor and a rotating group of members from their church came most evenings to pray out loud for the girl. Although we insisted, successfully, that the church group leave the room when we came, we had no medical basis for demanding that the mother leave us alone with her daughter.

When we talked with her in her mother's presence, Britney kept her eyes on her mother and let her do the talking. We could not learn from Britney directly how she felt about her illness or ongoing treatments. Instead, her mother said she wanted the treatments, and Britney nodded. When we queried Britney—gently, we thought—about how she imagined her future, she looked at her mother, who said her daughter expected God to save her, and Britney nodded. As we had no idea what her mother had told Britney about the value of the transfusions or her prognosis, we did not know how to interpret the nods. Once, when her mother left for an hour or so, the nurses alerted us that Britney was alone and we came by. I would like to report that we were able to talk with her, but she appeared to be sleeping deeply and we did not wake her up.

TRADITIONAL BIOETHICS
MAY NOT BE ENOUGH

Bioethics, the current term for what used to be known as *medical ethics*, gained its name and professional configuration during the early 1970s. I was in medical school then, and, like many fellow students and faculty, I was excited about its potential to guide day-to-day medical practice and clinical research. I still am. What I and others failed to appreciate then was that an ethicist or ethics committee's administrative situation within a hospital often constrains its ability to advocate for patient welfare. Early leaders of the field decided that bedside ethics would flourish within medical institutions only if ethicists and their committees adopted an educational and advisory role, not a regulatory one. Ethics committees were not to look at issues of patient welfare per se, but rather to offer educational programs and issue advisory opinions concerning ethical principles relevant to particular dilemmas. One result is that situations like Britney's may go on unless someone requests consultation with the ethics committee. Even then, hospital ethics committees do not issue orders, as do physicians when they prescribe an antibiotic. Nor do they set standards or provide oversight for patient welfare, as do their counterparts tasked with overseeing the welfare of animals used in medical research.

For Britney's situation, our committee recommended that her physicians authorize no more transfusions but proceed with comfort measures, including hospice, which is what they wanted, too. When they met with Britney's mother to discuss her daughter's care, however, her mother rejected their plan, picked up her daughter, and walked out. Anticipating this might happen, her doctors had already alerted regional blood banks of Britney's condition and her mother's potential response of going elsewhere for more transfusions. I was told that Britney died at home a short while later, as no hospital or blood bank would comply with her mother's demands. Her mother would not accept hospice care for her daughter at home or in the hospital.

Feeble communication among patients, families, and doctors lies behind most requests for consultations with hospital ethics committees. Usually, when an ethics committee meets with the various parties in settings that encourage active listening for all voices, the disputes can be resolved. Earlier on in this particular story, someone might have been able to engage Britney's father, and through him her mother and her pastor, but the family had fractured. We had hoped her pastor might function as a bridge, as clergy often do when relations turn fractious, but his theology was even stricter than her mother's, and he refused. Indeed, Britney's mother and pastor insisted on placing themselves on one side of what they imagined to be an existential abyss with her doctors and the hospital on the other.

Of the several thousand very sick people I have been involved with, the degree and extent of Britney's misery stand out. As her ordeal wore on—and her mother's resolve for additional treatment stiffened—no amount of thoughtful communication could have bridged the chasm between the secular outlook of her doctors and hospital and the absolutist theology of her mother. They simply are not compatible. In order to have a functioning bioethics as it is presently configured, one needs a modicum of reasonableness and trust in the goodness of ordinary humanity, two staples that disappear early in the Sturm und Drang of apocalyptic religion. Otherwise, one needs reliable administrative mechanisms to assure that extreme therapies are not undertaken without careful appraisal of their consequence for the patient's overall welfare.

Suppose one or another of Britney's doctors had recognized and accepted that incompatibility earlier in her illness, perhaps during a discussion with her family about the wisdom of amputating her lower pelvis. After considering her prognosis and the consequences of such a maiming for her ongoing life, suppose her surgeon and oncologist had told her parents they would not do the procedure because they thought it not in Britney's best interest. If they took that position, then to be complete and not leave Britney and her parents feeling abandoned, they would also have been obliged to outline more modest measures that might help her. One team actually tried that approach with her mother, which she rejected in favor of taking Britney elsewhere, where she persuaded another group to do the surgery.

What accounts for physicians' willingness to perform interventions against our better medical judgment? In medical hallways, doctors frequently cite fear of litigation, a fear some hospital attorneys second. To my knowledge, however, no physician has been successfully sued for not doing something he reasonably determined to be futile or against his better judgment, provided he did not then abandon the patient. Nonetheless, many of us, including myself on occasion, have acceded to patient demands for treatments we thought not indicated by the underlying condition. When the stakes are small—a parent's adamant request for an antibiotic for his febrile child who probably has a virus and needs only acetaminophen and fluids—a physician's willingness to accede and thereby have a "satisfied patient" seems a minor lapse.

As anyone who has cared for young children knows, we adults have limited access to the mysteries of their being. Our imaginations try to go there, and some excellent psychological studies approach their inner world, but we cannot experience it, as we can our own and other adult psyches, with a true sense of understanding. We know for certain, though, that there are major differences between children and adults. Psychological studies of the inner world of dying children repeatedly confirm my own impression that children up to the age of twelve or so tend to imagine death with less fear than adults do, especially if they have been very ill for a long time.

But that doesn't mean children with serious chronic illnesses do not want to know what is going on. In the mid-1970s a sociology graduate student, Myra Bluebond Langer, decided to spend time in a pediatric cancer unit. Instead of finding what she anticipated—open and clear communication among doctors, parents, and children—she observed elaborate intrigues. Doctors and parents talked with each other with some candor, but neither group talked much with the children. Meanwhile the children, determined to know what was going on, devised clever tactics to get in the loop. Adopting a "capture the flag'" approach, some teams designated lookouts and runners to steal the paper charts off the unit trolley and run them back to their beds for flashlight inspection under the bedcovers, the more literate interpreting for the less. Another team, inspired by Watergate perhaps, figured out how to put tape recorders in conference rooms and operate them remotely so as to record what the adults said about them in their endless conferences. All of this made for moments of high adventure, though I expect the moments did not assuage their despair at being excluded from discussions with their parents and doctors about what really mattered. Surrounded by adults, the children were nonetheless dying privately.

ETHICS AND CHILDREN'S VOICES

Whatever children may experience or imagine in sickness and in health, the historical reality is that their voices have counted for little in Western ethics. The Greek philosophers and healers who joined ethics and healing during the fourth century B.C.E. discussed appropriate conduct, their definition of ethics, in terms of adults, not children, and "free" adults at that. In terms of formal ethical principles, children, at least in Western philosophy, have mostly existed in an ethical shadowland where they are sometimes perceived as persons, albeit in junior form, and at other times as akin to property. When physicians and philosophers considered the moral status of children from the eighteenth century into the early twentieth, they paid little attention to children's consent for any aspect of their lives. Instead, they spent considerable effort discriminating between "public" children in orphanages, who were treated as public property, and children who live privately with their parents and were, by logical extension, private property. John Locke, so respected by America's founders for his philosophy of consent, recommended putting very young children to work in his model poorhouse of the early Enlightenment. After Edward Jenner first tested his smallpox vaccine on some children, including his own son, his vaccine was tried in Philadelphia in 1802 on forty-eight "public" children under the care of the director of a poorhouse.

Americans in the Victorian era, fond as they were of establishing institutions for the moral improvement of society, established the first American Society for the Prevention of Cruelty to Children in New York City in 1875, which was nine years after reformers established the New York Society for the Prevention of Cruelty to Animals. But Victorian versions of cruelty to children were not ours, for their values and laws still considered all children to be parental property in many respects, and potential income-producing property at that. Indeed, in the United States from the late 1800s into the early twentieth century, in low-income households a larger percentage of children from age ten onward worked outside the family home than the percentage of mothers who worked outside the home. Moreover, children represented a disproportionate percentage of the workforce in some dangerous occupations that benefited from small bodies and tiny fingers. In Southern textile mills that developed after the Civil War, for example, one-third of the workers were children between ten and thirteen years of age. And the parents tended to pocket their kids' earnings. The federal government did not significantly restrict child labor in the United States until the Great Depression of the 1930s, and then it was with the primary intention of opening up jobs for adults. (But then, who do we think makes many of our imported "hand-knotted" rugs today?)

For a moment after World War II, it seemed as though the ethical status of children might gain sustained attention. Revelations of Nazi medical atrocities, including those against children, during the Nuremberg Trials stimulated widespread resolve to establish a universal code of medical ethics. The 1947 Nuremberg code of medical ethics, however, like the American Medical Association code it was modeled on, did not discuss pediatric care or research. Instead, both codes, *pace* Locke, focused on consent: to do ethical research, investigators must obtain full voluntary consent from all persons participating in the research. But children then, as now, did not possess legal rights of consent, which means that the requirement, if taken literally, would have effectively excluded children from participating in research. When the public health stakes became high and a therapy looked promising, such as the Salk vaccine for the early 1950s polio epidemics, government, foundation, and medical leaders developed detailed consent forms for parents to sign on behalf of the hundreds of thousands of children undergoing vaccine trials. (They tried Salk's first virus vaccine earlier,without written parental consent, on a few thousand "public" children housed in state institutions.)

Other than testing vaccines on children, however, medical investigators well into the 1990s conducted relatively few randomized and double-blind drug trials—an epistemological gold standard—on children, and many of the existing ones included too few children to be persuasive. In a way no one intended, an ethical shadowland for children has become a scientific shadowland as well. During the past fifty years, pills for everything have proliferated, and treatment regimes for serious diseases, such as cancer, have become ever more aggressive. But most of these pills and regimes derive from research conducted on adults in middle life, not on young children. Children's bodies function differently from adult ones in important ways. Absent specific knowledge of how children might react differently from adults to a given treatment, we simply adjust dosages downward to reflect children's lower weight. But mere dose adjustment, while necessary, may still prove insufficient.

As with clinical research with children, those on life's other shore—the very elderly—also have been making do with many medicines that have never been specifically tested for suitability in *their* bodies. Although most adult bodies, gender differences aside, tend to metabolize substances in similar ways during their middle decades, those of the very elderly become more idiosyncratic. Yet comparatively few people over seventy-five participate in clinical trials, even though they tend to consume large numbers of medicines. The lack of knowledge about how a specific medicine that has been tested on groups with a median age of forty-five may behave in a seventy-five-year-old leads to frequent untoward reactions.

Early in my career, when chemotherapy with wide-acting cellular poisons demonstrated promise in treating some adult cancers, I spent time with Davey, a five-year-old boy with an invasive solid cancer who was being given one of the new agents. Because little research on the use of such agents had been conducted in young children, no one anticipated that the treatment would turn out to be worse than the disease. He died not of cancer, which seemed to have gone into remission if not been cured, but from the effects of the cellular poison on his heart. Should Davey not have received the treatment? Beyond familiarizing themselves sufficiently with the potential risks of the treatment *for him* and adequately informing his mother of them—which I hope they did—his physicians' ability to foresee his reaction through use of statistics based on other children's experiences with the medicine was limited.

Current ethical guidelines for pediatric research and treatment acknowledge the value of children's voices, though the extent to which the guidelines are followed in practice remains questionable. The American Academy of Pediatrics, for example, now recommends gaining a child's assent when it is possible and prudent. Institutional review boards, the local hospital bodies that administer clinical drug trials according to federal regulations, sometimes require pediatric researchers to obtain assent from their pediatric research subjects. Still, parents' wishes generally trump their children's.

MOTHERS AND BABIES

With the exceptions of physical abuse, the 1984 federal regulations governing the care of disabled infants (see below), and teens with sexual issues, the actual voices of children continue to count for little compared to their parents'. Paradoxically, however, the imagined voice of an "unborn child," an arcane phrase prior to the culture war that erupted around *Roe* v. *Wade*, has come to count for more. Indeed, in some settings, this imputed voice, imperceptible to human ears, may be deemed louder than that of the prospective mother whose body contains it. At the same time, today's prospective mother, in comparison to *her* mother, has a great deal more latitude to determine when and what kind of "unborn voice" she might carry, thanks to genetic screening and assisted reproduction technologies. Debates and the occasional public violence that have occurred around these developments tend to share one common feature: all parties present their positions in moral terms. Indeed, the fervent present their positions as zero-sum situations in which only one party can be right. While moral philosophy has always addressed tensions between duty and freedom, shifts in the *aesthetic* perception of human gestation may be an important generator of the rhetorical extremes that fill the air around pregnant women and their potential babies.

Prior to the 1960s, popular culture usually portrayed a pregnant woman and her fetus from the outside in. Glossy pregnancy guides from the 1950s, for example, are rife with large photos of expectant mothers beaming rhapsodically, followed by smaller line drawings of a developing fetus. One sees the expectant mother and imagines the fetus within; *she* always dominates the picture. I venture most people perceived the fetus as part of a woman's body, not as a creature in its own right. At that time, this was biologically true, as biomedicine had not yet created the reality of a fetus living outside the womb unless it was almost full-term.

Perceptions, if not biomedical reality, took a turn toward the fetus in 1965, when *Life* magazine published a series of color photographs by Lennart Nilsson that portrayed a developing human fetus inside its mother's womb. The images were close-ups— fetuses in the foreground with backgrounds left indeterminate. For the first time, one saw not the mother but the fetus, which of course demonstrated increasingly personlike features as the trimesters advanced. Shortly thereafter, the full series appeared in book form to wide acclaim, and its current edition remains a best-seller in its category. In terms of popular culture, the fetus had come into its own, a shift in moral status amplified subsequently by routine use of sonograms.

If *Life*'s splashy debut of the fetus as a miniperson profoundly affected popular perceptions about early human life, which is how the portfolio was celebrated at the time, the emergence in the early 1960s of "the Pill" from the lab into the world shifted not only perceptions, but life in the quotidian for millions of women. Some young women in Boston went further and expressed determination to take charge of their bodily care. In 1973 they published *Our Bodies, Ourselves*, a popular self-help guide by and for women of reproductive years that is still in print. In 1973 a conflicted U.S. Supreme Court decriminalized most intentional abortions, a decision that opened one front of the cultural war in which we are enmeshed today.

In 1971 a conflict over the plight of a single newborn had helped persuade one family—the political Kennedys—and the Jesuit leader of Georgetown University—that bioethics deserved their serious support. Their response to the fate of that infant, who came to be known as Baby Doe, helps explain why American society, including its medicine and ethics, cannot seem to reach a consensus about the moral status of children, born and unborn. Born at Johns Hopkins Hospital, the infant was the first of several Baby Does whose treatment provoked medical, ethical, and then legal disputes that stimulated federal regulations of the Reagan era and continue to direct how parents, doctors, and hospitals approach all newborns today.

When Baby Doe's mother became pregnant, amniocentesis and sonograms were not in the picture. If a pregnancy felt more or less right and went to or near to full term, everyone anticipated a thriving newborn. But Baby Doe was born with duodenal atresia, an intestinal obstruction that must be surgically corrected for survival. Although the condition is not common, it is not uncommon; more important, surgeons can correct it easily and with almost 100 percent success rates. This is what Baby Doe's Johns Hopkins surgeons proposed to do. Yet the parents said no, and left their baby for Hopkins staff to deal with. During the next fifteen days, Baby Doe's nurses and doctors placed him in a room by himself—his screams in the regular nursery quickly becoming unbearable—and witnessed his death by dehydration.

This was not the first baby with duodenal atresia abandoned by its parents to such a fate at Hopkins. A similar situation at the hospital three years earlier prompted Robert Cooke, then chair of Pediatrics, to seek a court order mandating the surgery, but the court declined, determining instead that the parents had the right to make that decision. Indeed, as Baby Doe lay dying, Norm Fost, Cooke's chief resident, went to the Hopkins records room and found six other contemporary examples of the same situation: newborns with duodenal atresia whose parents rejected medical advice and left their babies to die. (Baby Doe's pediatric intern, the late Bill Bartholome, subsequently told me he hated himself for participating in this. In fact, he said that the experience drove him into ethics, which he left Hopkins to study at Harvard Divinity School. Subsequently, Bill became a distinguished pediatrician and eloquent advocate for the rights of children. Ditto for Norm Fost, who went into ethics and has devoted his career to advocating on behalf of the eight to ten million American children who have no medical insurance and are not eligible for Medicaid, as well as those who suffer more overt physical abuse in their families.)

Not content to continue down the same path again, Baby Doe's caregivers alerted the Kennedys and Georgetown of what was going on, and with Kennedy Foundation backing they made a movie about Baby Doe, *Who Shall Survive?*, that has been seen by more than a million people. The film, in which Bill Bartholome reenacted his behavior as the intern, reveals why, in fact, Baby Doe's parents refused lifesaving surgery for their newborn: in addition to duodenal atresia, Baby Doe was born with Down syndrome. His parents, a youngish professional couple, said they wanted a baby, but they didn't want *that*, a "Mongol," as people with Down's were then commonly called. Indeed, before he became "Baby Doe," he was referred to as "the Hopkins Mongol case."

The two phrases—*a baby with Down syndrome* and *the Mongol case*—evoke quite different perceptions. The former tugs at the heart—the baby is a person, above all—whereas the latter was intended to signify something subhuman. In those days the medical establishment perceived Baby Doe more or less as his parents had—a subhuman, a "Mongol case." According to a national survey of pediatricians and pediatric surgeons published in the wake of the Baby Doe case, which was duplicated by a similar survey in Massachusetts, 70 percent of respondents indicated that what the parents wanted was acceptable. Echoing what Fost had found when he looked into Hopkins records, Dr. Raymond Duff, a prominent Yale pediatrician, reported in an article for *The New England Journal of Medicine* that over a two-year period, one in five deaths in the Yale–New Haven Hospital nursery resulted from the deliberate withholding of standard medical treatment for children with Down syndrome and other relatively modest disabilities, as well as for newborns so congenitally impaired they had little prospect of a long or meaningful life. Duff interpreted such hospital staff behavior differently from Fost, however. In the article's last paragraph he asserted: "If what we did is illegal, then that shows that the law needs to be changed."

What Duff and others in medicine failed to perceive was that everyone does not share their view of what it means to be human or humane. Just as *Roe* v. *Wade* started to split the country, the presumption that doctors could—indeed ought—to police the boundaries of humanity and collude with like-minded parents in sleight-of-hand eugenics provoked a backlash, of which the rhetoric of the "unborn child" is only one expression today. It took a few more Baby Doe legal cases, notably an Indiana Supreme Court decision in 1982, for Baby Doe's advocates to gain the upper hand, but when they did, they did their utmost to make sure their views prevailed. Their goal was to establish a default standard of care for disabled infants, which they have done. Because the regulations are tightly drawn, however, they leave little room for the exercise of prudence or *caritas*. Promoted enthusiastically by President Reagan, the rules are contained in amendments, commonly known among ethicists as the "Baby Doe" regulations, to the Child Abuse Prevention and Treatment Act of 1984. In place of individualized decision making for parents of newborns and their doctors, which for better *and* worse had been the standard, the amendments require state health departments to launch criminal investigations if they receive reports that doctors and nurses are not delivering maximal treatment to all infants under one year—even those with no chance of long-term survival—unless a physician can attest the infant is irreversibly comatose. Putting aside the irony that a president who championed diminished government was eager to insert the government into the most intimate recesses of family life, what have the regulations meant in practice? According to Norm Fost, they have been effective for newborns with Down's, as he knows of no child with Down syndrome who has died from the withholding of standard care since they came into effect.

IN THE NAME OF FREEDOM: WHAT "BABY DOE" REGULATIONS MAY MEAN FOR YOU

Reagan's regulatory mandate to treat maximally has also meant that too little treatment has given way to too much. For hopelessly impaired infants, its effects may well verge on the cruel. My colleague Loretta Kopelman, known in our field for her rigorous advocacy for shared decision making and patient's-best-interest standards in pediatrics, recently described an example of this to me. In the early 2000s, a ten-month-old boy, whom I shall call Joe, was admitted with acute kidney failure that his doctors could not explain or cure. In order to survive, he needed long-term kidney dialysis with a possible kidney transplant down the line. However, Joe was born with a severe and permanent structural brain abnormality that had rendered him capable of reacting only to painful stimuli. When his mother was not caring for Joe, she and her two daughters tended to his older brother, who had a less severe form of the brain abnormality and was also retarded as a consequence, though not as profoundly as Joe. If Joe lived with dialysis, it meant that he would be experiencing multiple painful needle sticks, among other intrusions, indefinitely. Who would pay the financial costs was another matter.

The pediatric residents taking care of Joe wanted to know from Dr. Kopelman if the "Baby Doe" regulations applied. They did. Does this make sense? If one agrees with the regulations, then would one also agree to nonstop burdensome treatments if Joe were six or sixteen or sixty-six when his kidneys failed? After all, if it was right to take Joe's doctors and parents out of the equation when Joe was ten months old on the grounds that they could not be trusted, what would be the reason for bringing them back in as he grew older?

Though the "Baby Doe" regulations apply in a strict sense only to infants under a year, their imperative to treat, treat, and treat will nevertheless carry on into childhood, as we have seen with Britney, and even beyond into advanced decades, as we have seen in other chapters. The hospital imperative to resuscitate anyone and everyone, hopelessly enfeebled or not, *unless* they have a recently signed Do Not Resuscitate (DNR) request, employs the same logic, and for some of the same reasons.

Regulations that tightly stipulate parameters of medical care for the enfeebled at either end of the life spectrum are, at best, a heavy-handed substitute for policies that seek to balance compassion, prudence, and a modicum of social trust. These qualities, along with an ability to listen, may be all we have. None of them alone fully resolves true dilemmas associated with treating very sick children—or dying adults—but in concert they can reveal falsity in the scenarios we sometimes construct for them and ourselves.

If we as a society took them seriously in terms of children's health, we would reinstitute good low-cost or no-cost nutritional programs in schools—millions of American children suffer malnourishment today—and provide sound preventive and acute health care for children. Instead, the school nurses who served the elementary schools of forty years ago have been eliminated in favor of governmental policies whose hypocrisy about "children's rights" verges on the obscene.

6

If This Is a Person

RYAN AND THE PILGRIM HOSPITAL, BOSTON, 1993

I was the staff emergency physician on duty one Saturday morning at the Pilgrim when an ambulance brought in an injured boy. Ryan, who was seventeen and went to high school in Boston's western suburbs, had woken up that morning eager to play soccer, which he did. On the way back from the game, though, a truck rammed the passenger side of the car in which he occupied the right front seat. Now he lay motionless in the Pilgrim's trauma room. What I saw was this: a fair-haired, pale teenage boy of a slender and wiry build, about five feet eight inches tall, who weighed around 125 pounds. He had bruises on his right forehead and temple, and his right upper arm and leg showed obvious deformities, though the skin was not broken. Ryan's airway, neck, chest, abdomen, and pelvis seemed normal on my emergency survey. Based on initial X-rays, Ryan's cervical spine looked good to me, and the orthopedic resident said the fractures—of an arm and a leg—did not require surgery and should heal well. X-rays of his chest, abdomen, and pelvis suggested that they were not injured, as did the absence of blood in his urine.

It was Ryan's brain that was the problem. Though his pupils responded normally to light, he moved his good arm in an unco-ordinated way when his chest was pinched. Despite breathing on his own and maintaining a stable pulse and blood pressure, he remained unconscious and unresponsive. Could a mass lesion—a bleed—have been causing Ryan's unresponsiveness? CAT scans of his skull showed no pool of blood or clots for the neurosur-geons to evacuate, and Ryan's ventricles and cisterns—the cavities in the brain that contain cerebral spinal fluid—were not obliter-ated, though two might have been compressed. (Compression of the ventricles is an ominous sign, especially when it is not caused by a discrete mass, for it suggests that a diffuse injury is causing the brain to swell. Too much swelling in a closed compartment like the skull frequently leads to irreversible brain damage or worse, the upper brain forcing the lower brain downward against bony protuberances inside the base of the skull, a situation that often leads to death if it is not halted promptly.) Although Ryan was breathing on his own and maintaining a decent level of blood oxygen, we intubated his trachea and put him on a ventilator in case his brain swelled. If the ventilator was set to stimulate his breathing slightly, the level of carbon dioxide in his blood would fall, and studies on patients with severe head injuries as well as an-imal studies suggest this would likely lower his intracranial pres-sure. We also elevated the head of Ryan's bed thirty degrees, and

I put an intravenous catheter in his left jugular vein to monitor his blood levels of carbon dioxide and oxygen. Our care was "supportive," and it did not feel like much.

We speculated that Ryan's brain had sustained a diffuse axonal injury. The back-and-forth collision of his head into solid parts of the car had profoundly, if subtly, damaged his brain's cortex, even as his brain stem was capable of directing his vital functions. An MRI would be able to detect focal abnormalities in his frontal and temporal lobes as well as in the corpus callosum, the structure that connects the right and left cerebral hemispheres. Ryan's family had not yet arrived, and I turned to other patients as he went for his MRI.

"Will he recover?" I asked the neurosurgical resident.

"Hard to say," he responded. "He's a teenager, so he'll probably do better than either an infant or adult, but we'll just have to see. It depends. His ventricles look a little compressed, not a good sign. About 40 percent with his injury die in the hospital."

What I knew about long-term outcomes for severely brain-injured people was that many apparent recoveries turned into tragedies, as about 40 percent end up in a persistent vegetative state (PVS), often after an initial lengthy coma. The resident suggested I call the organ transplant coordinator—"Better to start with the family early." To look at Ryan, relatively unmarked except for the forehead and temple bruises, one would not have perceived him to be at the end of his life. His skin was pink and warm and his breathing regular, and he looked asleep. Indeed, he looked very much like my oldest son, who was fifteen, slight and wiry, and devoted to soccer. I did not call the transplant coordinator.

About two hours had passed since Ryan arrived. He was back

from his MRI, though I had not yet seen it, and his family was waiting for news in the "Quiet Room." On the way to see them with a nurse, the transplant coordinator found us. Her position was new, part of the Pilgrim's push to become dominant in the Boston organ transplant "market." She wanted to come in with us to talk with the family, "After you do, of course, Dr. Martensen." I demurred; the timing was not right for this. I told the coordinator that Ryan was stable now; she could talk with the family in another setting later. But the coordinator, not pleased, switched into an earnest mode: "You *do* know, don't you, Dr. Martensen, that our new program involves early intervention in the ER. It's been shown to increase the harvest rate if we talk to the families early. I saw you at the presentation we did for your ER group."

Though I loathed her agricultural euphemism—*harvest* was the new buzzword in the transplant world—I thanked her for coming in on a Saturday. Then the nurse and I left her outside the door of the Quiet Room and went in to see Ryan's family. When we were all introduced to each other—they numbered fourteen or fifteen—we sat down. I talked about what had happened to Ryan.

"What should we do?" his parents asked the nurse and me.

"Talk to him," I said. "Talk to him as though he can hear you. We do not know his future, what his function will be. It may well take weeks to sort out." The ER was busy, and I left them as a priest came in.

Even as I continued seeing patients that day, what moved in and out of my mind were memories of another young man who went into prolonged coma twenty years earlier, while I was studying to become a doctor and *persistent vegetative state* was a new phrase in the medical vocabulary.

SUSPENDED ANIMATION: DARTMOUTH, 1973

Caleb was a teenager and breathing on a ventilator and I was a twenty-six-year-old medical student at Dartmouth when we first encountered each other in August 1973. He looked as though he were sleeping, and he had been that way for almost three months. His eyes used to open and close spontaneously two months earlier. But no movement since, just a flaccid paralysis. All Caleb's deep tendon reflexes—the doctor's tap below the kneecap—were gone. Talking to him or pinching him or giving him a whiff of ammonia elicited nothing. Indeed, only his pupils responded reflexively: when one shined a light in one pupil, it contracted, and so did the other. That, and the fact that his pupils maintained normal diameters, were probably the only good neurological signs Caleb had, for they showed his midbrain was working. In every way possible, though, he depended on critical care nurses, doctors, and machines. In the meantime, he was excreting and even growing. Caleb's puberty had just kicked in.

He was a big-boned youth, about six feet tall and weighing 170 pounds, preternaturally pale and with scattered pimples on his puffy face. Whenever I saw Caleb, I also saw his parents. He was their only child. Day in and day out and on most nights, one or the other stayed by his side in the small side room in the ICU where Caleb now lived. Their names were Stephan and Sofia, and like their son, they were big-boned with fair skin and dark hair and eyes. They might have been brother and sister, so alike did they look. Originally from Hungary, they had come to this country as newlyweds in 1956 to get away from the Russians. Caleb was conceived shortly after they arrived in Boston, which was why they had given him a New England–style name, not a Hungarian one. He would be a "true American." Since Caleb had come here, by which they meant the ICU, they had switched around their jobs—his with a nearby fire department and hers with the hospital food service—so that one or the other, and ideally both, could stay with their son. What else could they do?

Baffled, the doctors did not know what to tell Caleb's parents. They did not know when Caleb would come out of the coma— if in fact he was in a coma—nor did they know why he had fallen into the coma in the first place. They suspected he was experiencing an extreme case of Guillain-Barré syndrome. But no test existed then (or now) to rule Guillain-Barré in or out. Compared to a disease such as childhood diabetes, which has biochemical markers, the boundaries of a syndrome, whether severe or mild, remain fuzzy by definition. Diagnosis of Guillain-Barré is suggestive and wholly clinical, which means it fits a picture composed of symptoms and signs that doctors can observe. Although almost everything about the course of Caleb's problems fit Guillain-Barré, Dartmouth's neurologists, an experienced group, had never seen or read about a patient with Guillain-Barré going into a coma before. Before Caleb had descended into coma, he had leg weakness, followed by weakness in his arms and facial muscles, followed by increasing paralysis, all symptoms typical of Guillain-Barré. Before Caleb had developed these symptoms, he had experienced a cold, which is also characteristic of the syndrome.

Guillain-Barré syndrome, which was named in 1916, is an example of the body's unpredictable reaction to an event, in Caleb's case most likely the recent cold. As the syndrome runs its course, it is as though the body becomes allergic to part of itself, which is why it is considered an autoimmune disorder. People with severe

Guillain-Barré become paralyzed when their own immune systems, rather than toxic proteins from some bacterial invader like tetanus or rabies, inflame their peripheral motor nerves at their intersections with muscle cells. Most of the time the inflammatory reaction is weak, sensory nerve roots are spared, and symptoms are mild and disappear over weeks. Sometimes, however, sensory nerves are affected, which is probably why Caleb reported numbness and tingling early on. In a percentage of the affected, Guillain-Barré paralyzes the muscles of the chest wall, and the patient may die. Nothing cures the syndrome, just as nothing cures tetanus; unlike tetanus, however, there is no vaccine for Guillain-Barré. But if Caleb did have Guillain-Barré, his brain was likely functioning, for the syndrome is not thought to involve neurons in the central nervous system. He would be sensing and thinking, but his total paralysis would prevent an observer from knowing for certain that he was. He would exist in a frightening (and rare) carapace, in which he could feel and sense and think but be incapable of expressing anything.

Was Caleb, in his paralyzed state and seemingly asleep, still capable of perceiving the external world? Not knowing what he might or might not be perceiving, his doctors told his parents and nurses that they should just talk to him in ordinary ways. This meant having technical discussions out of Caleb's earshot on the off chance that he might hear and be disturbed.

Sofia and Stephan took this to mean they should keep Caleb up on his regular interests—TV's *Twilight Zone* and the Red Sox being the principal ones. They turned on the TV and radio when either was being broadcast, and they read him the sports pages from *The Boston Globe* and most of *Sports Illustrated*, spiced with *Popular Mechanics* and the occasional car magazine. Caleb's best friend from school came by often and told him jokes and what everyone was up to. And so the weeks passed. As the summer flowed on and Caleb remained in a coma, his parents would start talking about Caleb finishing high school and going to college before their voices trailed off. All of us were concerned that he was not waking up. Since an extended coma was not typical of Guillain-Barré, we had no idea if, or when, Caleb might reenter the regular world. *When will Caleb wake up?* became, without anyone ever mentioning it, *Will Caleb wake up?* No one wanted to put the question in words, but one could see the shift in everyone's face. By September, the question of his future had become acute.

Neurologists were and are brilliant examiners, but before CAT scans (and then MRIs and PET scans), they gained most of their knowledge not by studying images of functioning brains, but through the close observation of people's exteriors, awareness, and capacities. Simple X-rays have never been very good for delineating subtle aspects of soft tissues, especially when a process is diffuse. Unlike today, when a PET scan can light up exactly which part of the brain is active for a Buddhist doing a specific type of meditation, neurologists then had no way of directly visualizing what brains were doing. For generations they relied instead on questions and taps and tests of someone's motor and sensory functions and mental states to correlate seemingly tiny signs of neurological dysfunction with diseases whose outer signs might otherwise have remained obscure. Autopsies, not images of living brains, provided the diagnostic confirmation.

Although Dartmouth was then about to install a CAT scanner, one of the nation's first, we could not have slid Caleb into its narrow chamber because we could not have maintained his ventilation when he was inside. Electrical recordings—EEGs—of the brain's activity often provided useful information, but their analysis then was not as refined as it is today, especially in comalike states that had been going on for a while. We performed EEGs on Caleb regularly, but they were not specific for anything, displaying instead only diffuse slowing and dampened amplitudes consistent with someone on sedatives. Caleb's neurologists talked about doing a brain biopsy on him, but ruled it out because of the risks. Was his brain functioning or not? And if so, was his cortex—the part we have come to think of as containing our identity as persons—working? We simply could not tell.

We students began to wonder if Caleb could be in what we were just starting to hear about, a "persistent vegetative state." Dr. Fred Plum, the coauthor of a short text on stupor and coma that we all relied upon, was also coauthor, with Dr. B. Jennett, of this new phrase. Spurred by our teachers, we mused upon Caleb's state in light of Dr. Plum's definition. As in his previous writing on stupor and coma, Dr. Plum was pithy in his original 1972 article about PVS in *The Lancet*: "New methods of treatment may, by prolonging the lives of patients with conditions which were formerly fatal, result in situations never previously encountered." He continued, "Few would dispute that in this condition the cerebral cortex is out of action." In other words, the lower brain could be working, as Caleb's pupillary reactions demonstrated, but the brain's upper regions, its cortex or cerebral hemispheres, might be persistently nonfunctional. As Drs. Plum and Jennett emphasized, determination of PVS was clinical. No single test or set of tests could confirm it, and in those days no consensus existed about its timeline—the point when one could say someone was not in a coma but persistently vegetative. PVS was simply too new for anyone to know anything definitive about it.

Could this be our Caleb? We—all of us medical students, nurses, doctors, technicians, and his family and friends who spent time by his heaving ventilator—moved through our days on the edge of despair about him, and perhaps Caleb despaired, too. From the pediatric clerkship I moved on to surgery and anesthesia, but in free moments I continued to circle back to the ICU to see Caleb and his parents. A number of other students who spent time with them also did so. Our little "Caleb group" sometimes gathered at his bedside at the end of the day. We would watch him and look for signs. Stephan and Sofia still read to him each day, still turned on the TV, and still talked to him about the Red Sox, but their voices became increasingly listless.

During those gray winter days, Caleb's mother and father began to notice something. When they entered the room and started talking to him, he seemed different, more alert somehow, though they could not put their finger on how. Then, one morning in late January, approximately nine months after Caleb was first admitted into the emergency room, one of the Caleb group, an intern, hurried over at lunch to say that Caleb's fingers and toes were twitching. Caleb had moved! His parents, usually so stolid, were overwhelmed. Leaning forward earnestly, they whispered to us that they had hoped against hope for this moment and now they were afraid to hope for too much. As word got around the hospital, more of us sought out Caleb's bedside, so many that the nurses began enforcing the visitor limit. Two days after he twitched his fingers, Caleb began moving his arms with purpose; a couple of days later he moved his legs. Along the way he experienced that immensely poignant moment when he opened his eyes and looked around. It was late at night, and only his parents were there. He saw them! He knew them! It was enough for them:

their stolidity gave way to broad smiles when I saw them the next day. No longer content to sit still on either side of his bed, they caressed his face with its new peach fuzz and asked everyone, "What should we do now to help?"

Within a week Caleb no longer needed a ventilator, though it stayed in the room in case he relapsed, as some with Guillain-Barré were known to do. And then he began talking. "What happened to me?" he kept asking his mom and dad. Like many other patients who go into coma and recover, he had little idea of time. He still thought it was early spring, that he had been "out" for maybe a couple of weeks. He remembered that the Red Sox had swept a four-game series with the Yankees over the Fourth of July, and that it had happened on the Yankees' turf. But Boston's glorious run had happened long after Caleb's accident. Although he had appeared to be unconscious, he had actually been hearing and understanding some things around him. He also remembered his mother crying one day, but he had no idea when. Fortunately, like many who experience severe trauma or go into a coma and then come out, he had little memory of any significant pain. What mattered to him most, he said, was getting back on his feet and eating. A month after he twitched, he was home, nicking himself with his new razor and bemoaning his loss of a school year. On his follow-up visits to the pediatric clinic that I managed to attend, Caleb exhibited no cognitive deficits. Aside from occasional numbness and tingling in his fingers, he said he felt fine. According to our new CAT scanner, whose tube Caleb was now able to enter, his brain showed no atrophy or loss of cortical mass, which is typical in PVS. His muscle conduction studies and an EEG were normal.

Exactly what had happened to Caleb remains unclear. After an extensive review of his case and the world literature, his neurologists finally stayed with their midsummer diagnosis, which was that Caleb had endured an extreme form of Guillain-Barré syndrome complicated by a low-level autoimmune inflammation of his brain whose origins remained a mystery.

Although Caleb was never in PVS, he might easily have been. If he had gone into respiratory arrest at home or on the pediatric ward, where the hospital had originally thought to place him instead of the ICU, his brain might have spent several minutes without oxygen before he was resuscitated. The very intervention that had kept him alive—an emergency intubation of his airway and mechanical ventilation—would have served to get him back only to the partial life of someone who was persistently vegetative. It struck us students as curious that if that had occurred, we might not have been able to tell the difference for months.

ENCOUNTERING RYAN'S FATHER

Three weeks after that initial Saturday with Ryan, I ran into Ryan's father in the Pilgrim's lobby. The previous week Ryan had seemed to squeeze his father's finger when he had stroked his hand. There had been no purposeful movement since. The organ donation people had been by again, "just to have another chat" with the parents. Ryan continued to maintain his vital functions, and his fractures showed signs of healing on X-rays. The hospital's discharge planner was preparing his transfer to a chronic care facility.

"What are Ryan's chances?" his father asked me.

"I don't know what his chances are right now," I said. "The neurologists and neurosurgeons will have a much better idea."

"What do you think we should do?"

"Stay by your son," I said. "Keep talking to him. It's only been a few weeks since the injury. A recent study of people in comas who subsequently recovered showed that some of them remember bedside conversations. Talk to Ryan as though he is aware, even though he may not be. The study didn't explore people with injuries like your son's, but it's possible that at some deep level he may be aware." I added that the longer Ryan remained unresponsive, the less likely it was that he would recover significant function, though we did not really know.

"And if he doesn't wake up?" Ryan's father asked.

At one of our weekly ER physician staff meetings not long thereafter, Dr. Meldrum, our new ER director, brought in the transplant coordinator to give us an update on the program in relation to the ER. She reminded us that the Pilgrim had been a pioneer in transplant surgery. She really needed us "to talk with those families." The Pilgrim had been losing "market share" to Mass General and the Lahey Clinic in this area. As she wound up her talk, she noted that some of us had not been requesting her presence as early as we might. She and Dr. Meldrum would like us to call her at *any* time—a pause as she provided us with her cell phone number and Meldrum nodded—when patients with major trauma looked as though they might not survive.

During the Q&A that followed her presentation, I raised my hand. Transplants are great, I said. But isn't our mission in the ER to spend all our efforts on supporting the life of our patients? Aren't families experiencing enough shock at the news that their loved one has a serious, maybe fatal injury? Can't she wait until a little later than inside the ER to talk with families? For one thing, it puts us ER physicians in an awkward role with the families. How can they be sure we are doing our utmost for their loved one as we deliver the news, if we quickly switch to talk with them about organ donation? I know a number of my colleagues shared these views, but none of them spoke. She and Dr. Meldrum did not respond directly, but their body language suggested my queries were not the response they hoped to receive.

What she and Dr. Meldrum did not say was that major transplant operations, as a colleague at another medical school recently put it, have become the "financial lifeblood" of academic hospitals. Technically, hospitals like the Pilgrim and many nonacademic community hospitals in America are nonprofit, though many have converted to for-profit status by selling themselves to major Wall Street "health care" corporations. The Pilgrim, though, seems determined to remain, as it always has been, a nonprofit teaching and research hospital at the core of Harvard Medical School's clinical activities. Nonetheless, the "operating surpluses" generated by expensive procedures that are well insured—and nothing surpasses major organ transplants in this regard—can mean the difference between red and black on a hospital's annual report. A successful program can fill up surgical ICUs and even support the development of new ones.

And the Pilgrim, like many academic hospitals in this era, had stated repeatedly that it needed increased revenues. Although it was and is one of the wealthiest hospitals in the world, with hundreds of millions of dollars in its endowment and numerous well-funded research programs, in the early 1990s it was losing money on an operating basis. The hallway scuttlebutt in those years was that it was dipping into capital for the first time to make ends meet. Which was why the hospital was undertaking major "marketing initiatives" in many areas, with increased performance of major organ transplants at the top of the list.

What the Pilgrim's leadership did not say was that its financial shortfalls, like those of Boston's other prestigious hospitals, were largely of its own making. Clustered as they are around Harvard Medical School (except for Mass General, which is across town), each had behaved as a fiefdom unto itself, giving little thought to the overall need for new medical facilities in Boston in the era of managed care. Instead, each proliferated; at the moment, all of the hospitals lined up next to Harvard were dramatically expanding their outpatient capacities and adding amenities like valet parking to lure "customers" from affluent suburbs. In the meantime, inner-city patients with penetrating trauma, the stuff of the knife and gun clubs of jobless young adults, were shunted when possible to Boston City, which is a public facility. Penetrating trauma does not pay.

During our annual reviews that year from Dr. Meldrum, a number of us ER doctors heard that we were not being sufficiently supportive of the hospital, especially in marketing. In our individual meeting, Meldrum told me to "get with the program." "Really?" I responded. My feedback from patients had been pretty good, I reminded him, not to mention feedback from fellow physicians. I had also managed to publish quite a bit. "That's not what I'm talking about," he continued. He mentioned that the Pilgrim hoped to add a helicopter pad to its roof to attract the "blunt trauma" associated with vehicular injuries, the kind that Ryan experienced, as they are usually insured. (Auto insurance is mandatory in Massachusetts.) But first the Pilgrim must block its neighbor, Beth Israel Hospital, from getting *their* helicopter pad, which was why political consultants had been added to the Pilgrim's payroll.

Meldrum admonished me less than a hundred yards from where a Harvard committee in 1968 first agreed on a new criterion of death—"whole brain death"—as a substitute for death's traditional medical definition, which was cessation of cardiopulmonary function. A determination of "whole brain death," which soon became established as the legal criterion for death in all fifty states, requires physicians to document, among other things, complete cessation of electrical impulses from brain activity in the cortex and brain stem, as opposed to documenting a stopped heart. What is often overlooked in revisiting that moment is that the person who most promoted the new criterion, the anesthesiologist Henry Beecher, did so not to facilitate transplants, but rather to ameliorate the suffering of terminally ill patients receiving unrelenting treatments in ICUs. He reasoned that if it could be shown that their whole brains—cortex and brain stem included—were nonfunctional, then it was pointless, in fact harmful, to continue subjecting dying people to aggressive critical care.

We physicians work with patients one at a time, and in the ER we do so in a unique moral space—24/7, with no questions asked about immigration status, nor any requirement for ability to pay, and with every effort made for the well-being of that individual. Serving emergency patients is our end; for us they are not a means to something else. To consider an emergency patient in the context of a financial or utilitarian calculus regarding the transplant potential of his or her organs is not for the treating physicians to do. Moreover, at the time of severe brain injury or metabolic insult—the two general conditions that may lead to PVS—medical science has no reliably predictive tools to determine who may or may not end up in PVS or a minimally conscious state. Whatever we know about these conditions, we do know this: they only become apparent after months have elapsed, and even then physicians cannot definitively say who is vegetative and who is minimally conscious.

As PVS has become more common and the demand for organs from living donors grows, a number of bioethicists, notably those connected with active transplant programs, have echoed the arguments of some early *Lancet* editorials, albeit for a different reason. They argue that Harvard's 1968 definition of brain death should be expanded to include PVS. The critical biological feature of personhood, they maintain, is a functioning cerebral cortex. Absent that—as is the case by definition in PVS—they assume a person is alive in name only and would be better off dead.

During the time I was seeing Ryan, I worked half-time at the Pilgrim and half-time as a historian of medicine in other departments at Harvard. During a Harvard-MIT conference on culture, medicine, and personhood, anthropologists, philosophers, and historians from India, Brazil, Europe, and Boston shared our findings on the question of what makes a body a person. What my colleagues presented, and my own historical research has confirmed, is this: it is only in the West that we define the physiological spaces of personhood in terms of the cerebral cortex. Every other healing tradition—the great texts of traditional Chinese medicine, Hindu or Ayurvedic healing, Buddhism, and orally transmitted vernacular traditions—has tended to locate personhood in the soul and equated life with a beating heart. They understood what it is to be human and envisioned the human body differently from the ways we do. Their uncertainties about the dividing line between life and death of the body and person—and the duties and behavior codes that flow from their perceptions—reveal different aesthetic and moral imaginations.

Robert Desjarlais, an anthropologist with whom I worked at Harvard, spent two years among the Yolmo wa of north-central Nepal during the late 1980s. At the conference he noted the following:

Although the body is extremely important in the practical matters of illnesses, health, and everyday life, it is not especially bewildering to this Tibetan Buddhist people. It is often thought of as a kind of dwelling, composed of a loose collection of organs, which houses a set of psychological and spiritual forces. When the body is imbued with life, it is sacrosanct, but when the rnam-shes *departs, it is thought of as being "empty," a mere "bundle of discarded clothes," as one man puts it. While cremating a corpse in the hours following a death, then, the Yolmo wa treat it without undue reverence, handling it less like a sacred temple than a hollow bag of bones. They drink tea by its side, tug clothes off its frame, and carry it roughly to the cremation hill—where flesh and bones are "stuck" into the ground. While all this is going on, the soul, devoid of its corporeal abode, wanders as a person normally would, and returns home each day at dusk to eat with her family. But since the dead person lacks corporeal form, the family fails to see or hear her, and she soon leaves distressed and confused. During the next forty-nine days of funeral practices, family members and lamaic priests try to inform the deceased as to her status and to provide the best destination for her soul in a future life. Thus, in contrast to the modern West, it is the soul that does not know it is dead yet and prompts the most pressing of worries. The bottom line is that, for the Yolmo wa, it is the soul, rather than the body, that is most important.*

Even in the West, the idea that a well-functioning cerebral cortex is the sine qua non for full status as a human being does not stretch back as far in time as the founding of Harvard College. Which is why, if this new definition of death as whole brain death *or* PVS eventually prevails, I wonder how people two or three hundred years hence will regard this standard in terms of its justification for performing living donor transplants. Better technologies for failing organs will doubtless have arisen and supplanted transplants by then, so how will our successors interpret the ethics of what some propose to do now, which is to cut open people who appear to be living and take out their major organs, which kills them, to put their hearts, livers, and lungs in someone else?

Even before PVS gained its name in 1972, *The Lancet* published an editorial in 1970 entitled "Not Strive Officiously." It was about the social implications of prolonged medical attention for, among others, the "unconscious patient . . . sustained indefinitely in an unconscious state" and those in "vegetative states." The unnamed author wrote, "This is society's concern because of the high cost—notably in nursing skill—and the relatives' because of the protracted test to which they are submitted." The implication of the editorial was that public discussion of these issues would lead to medical policies that society might be able to accept. After noting the "infant with severe neurological abnormality," the "youngster with a crippling head injury," and those in "vegetative states," among others, as examples of human beings routinely subject to "unrelenting application of modern techniques," the author closed with the sentiment that "what counts is not the age at which someone dies but the quality of his life."

Then, a year later, *The Lancet* continued its existential musings with the publication of "Death of a Human Being," an editorial that questioned the personhood of those experiencing "neocortical death" and other severe neurological impairments. With PVS not yet named but its silhouette clearly in view, the editorialist wrote: "While one would agree that, with the total and irreversible cessation of brain function, the life of a human being has ceased, would it be any significant step further to say that if neocortical death is proved, the life of the human being has ceased to exist?" The leap had been made. For the writer, the sine qua non of human life was now not a beating heart or even a brain able to maintain basic bodily functions, but a vital cerebral cortex. According to this view, one was dead when in fact one could look very much alive: breathing, excreting, growing, menstruating perhaps—but not thinking or feeling or able to process sensations. Whereas whole brain death makes existence impossible for more than the very short term regardless of the level of technical medical support, neocortical death, as we know from Terri Schiavo and others, does not. Nonetheless, the writer suggested that existentially, they amount to the same thing.

Equally important, he was confident society would agree with his proposition. In his words:

> *Nevertheless, we may ask whether anyone would actually want his own vegetative existence to be artificially prolonged after the unequivocal diagnosis of any one of the states mentioned—whether brain death, cortical death, irreversible brain destruction, or permanent coma. Equally, who that knows the facts would want a close relative so supported? It is a dreadful decision, but the answer can hardly be in doubt.*

A few years later, in 1977, a prominent American physician, John Knowles, extended this new paradigm of humanity and projected it into the womb in an article entitled "The Responsibility of the Individual," which he published in *Daedalus*. Knowles, who served as a leader of Massachusetts General Hospital before heading the Rockefeller Foundation, discussed the need for pregnant women to use a then new technology, amniocentesis, to detect the fetal presence of Down syndrome. Knowles's overall focus in the article was on preventive medicine at the individual level. He assumed that if a woman knew her fetus had the genetic profile of Down syndrome, she would, of course, obtain an abortion. His tacit assumption was that any fetus with Down's was less than legitimately human and therefore should not enter the world. He presented his viewpoints as if they could meet no rational objection.

Like America's Founding Fathers, who often claimed Greco-Roman precedents for their new political theories, many scientists and physicians, not to mention ethicists, trace their approaches back to the Greeks, especially when they are talking about rationality and the human body. But the propositions Knowles and the *Lancet* editorialists advanced about what constitutes a person make truly novel claims. Although one can find continuities between ancient Greek notions of personhood and ours, one may be surprised at the thinness of Greek physiological literature concerning what we call "mental disability" today. The Greeks recognized dull-wittedness, but the subject did not seem to preoccupy them medically or socially. The Hippocratic texts, for example, discuss the condition of clubfoot in five places, but they make only one reference to congenital dull-wittedness. When Aristotle or Plato refers to congenital conditions or life stages that might result in loss of cognitive function, the organ of reference is the heart, not the brain. Nor did classical Greek thinkers automatically put intellectually dull people on humanity's margins. Instead, according to Plato at least, that space was reserved for "the most expert of calculators" who "hates, not loves, what his judgment pronounces to be noble or good." In other words, Plato found unvirtuous knowledge to be meaningless, but not necessarily dull-wittedness. The unwise clever were the biggest fools, he maintained; it was they who needed to be removed for remedial training so that they could be "styled wise."

So how was I to respond to Ryan's father as he contemplated his son's fate? We sat down together in the lobby, and I told him what I knew of the science at that time. If Ryan was in PVS, which could not be determined so soon, then his outlook was grim. Since he was on the cusp of adulthood, I mentioned the outcome studies of adults who entered PVS due to traumatic brain injury. Ryan's chances of making it for a year and coming out with some function and awareness were a little better than one in four. The longer he remained unresponsive, the worse his long-term prospects, with 95 percent of those dying within five years of its diagnosis. After a year in PVS, though, anyone who "recovers" without fail demonstrates severe disabilities of function and awareness. Ryan's father said his son's current physicians had told him more or less the same. He wept—and I did, too.

About Ryan's status as an organ donor, which was the question behind his father's question, I kept quiet. Not only do I not know the answer, I doubt that medicine and its modern ethics can generate a universal one. Who are we in biomedicine to claim that we know the meaning of human identity? Despite the elucidation of biological mechanisms that have proven to be universal in humans, biomedical formulations of personhood are just one of many that have crossed and will continue to cross the world's stage. So how can contemporary physicians legitimately claim absolute privilege in determining the boundaries of personhood, including when it ends? When biomedical leaders maintain that their instrumental rationality is the only legitimate means of experiencing the world, including illness and disability, I would argue they step outside medicine's boundaries to the verge of scientistic imperialism.

Even within medicine's legitimate boundaries, physicians and ethicists who maintain that those living in PVS and related states are mere bodies and not persons have their work cut out for them. Less is known about PVS and related diagnostic categories, such as minimal consciousness, than they let on. For example, one recent plausible study suggests that as many as 30 percent of those in PVS are minimally conscious; that is, they are aware of and respond in limited ways to human interactions. Are we ready to say with absolute confidence that *their* lives as they are living them have no worth?

Even with fresh donors whose brains are deemed to be wholly dead, transplant physicians commence their "harvests" of the "dead" person's parts by administering general anesthesia. But why do they need to do so if the brain-dead person is, in fact, dead? A British anesthesiologist faced the issue head-on in a 1999 letter to the *Journal of the Royal Society of Medicine*: "The greatest misconception is that the donor will be dead in any ordinary sense of the word." As the anthropologist Lesley Sharp recently noted (and as I have witnessed): "A brain-dead body [that has not been anesthetized] will move in a lifelike way when nerves are pinched or cut. [It] may seem to shrug or kick or even signal."

As a society we need to engage in reasonable discussions about how we respond ethically, legally, and financially to the challenges posed by PVS and minimally conscious states. At a minimum, the interested parties, especially the transplant lobby, should candidly disclose their philosophical assumptions, financial interests, and lacunae in scientific understanding of brain death, cortical and whole. Organ transplantation is an invaluable way to extend life at present. But constructing fictions about some of its underlying realities renders sordid what ought to be resolved in clear light.

I do not know what happened to Ryan; I wish I did. Not long after my review with Dr. Meldrum, nine of the fourteen other ER physicians and I left the Pilgrim, and the rest of our original group have since left or now work elsewhere within Harvard. Meanwhile, I wonder what would have happened to Caleb if he had come to the hospital in 2008 instead of 1973. Suppose eight months had passed and he was ventilator-dependent and diagnosed with PVS. Should the hospital's transplant marketers exert subtle pressure on Sofia and Stephan to submit their son for "harvesting"? Although it is a question that cannot be answered, it is one worth thinking about.

7

Life in the Narrows

Readers of these pages have likely enjoyed broad latitude in choosing their work, partners, and other contours of their lives. Until something bad happened to them, most of the people I have described so far—Ryan, hit by a car; Mike, with his terminal cancer; Ellen's experience of acute respiratory failure; and Eliza, with her octogenarian heart failure—enjoyed similar latitude. In this chapter I bring together a few people who have not been so fortunate. Unlike us, they must confine themselves to constricted paths that vary little. Their anguish tends not to be temporary, but recurrent. Their circumstances vary considerably, so much so that at first glance their commonality may not be apparent. What they share—and what sets them apart from most of us, I venture—is the level of their day-to-day vulnerability to social factors and cultural values. For one reason or another, they have had to depend on others for their basic welfare much more than most of us do. When others recognize their situations and provide support, their lives, dauntingly narrow when glimpsed from the outside, seem to gain amplitude. When others turn on them or the system leaves them little room, the consequences, inside and outside, may be dire.

I offer this chapter as a witness to what has gone on and will likely continue for those who live in the narrows, and desperately so. If I did not include them, this book would not be complete. When I decided to become a doctor in the 1970s, I never expected to practice in an America where the dire has become an everyday experience for so many. I began as an optimist in an optimistic time, at least in health care. For the past thirty years, however, life has not gotten better for our most vulnerable. Through Democratic and Republican administrations alike, compassion has been scarce, despite political and commercial expressions to the contrary. Though our health care approaches squander billions on extravagant treatment regimes that end up accomplishing little, as a society we refuse to adopt the small, even tiny, adjustments that could easily reduce the clawing uncertainties that now degrade millions.

Although I am close to despair about America's *public* imagination concerning our obligations to the needy and vulnerable, I take heart from what families routinely do on their own.

ACCEPTANCE

Nate Winstead and I first met around thirty years ago, when I left my small Michigan town for New England and a school classmate, one of his younger siblings, introduced me to his family. Since then we have all stayed in touch. Nate and I have become especially close, as we work together at the same hospital. He doesn't drive, so sometimes on warm Saturdays I take him up to his parents' place on Boston's North Shore for the day and visit with his relatives before dropping him off. Now Nate is turning fifty, and if I don't step on it, I'll be late for his party. My assignment is to pick up Mary, who helped raise him and who now lives with her sister a few miles north of Boston. Nate likes to start on time. "Schedule, Rob," he's said to me more than once. "Keeping on schedule very important, Rob." Alas, the road to Mary's has clogged up.

If it were up to Nate, we'd be celebrating out on the North Shore, where he grew up and where he feels most at home. "But then your hospital friends wouldn't come, Nate," his mother pointed out. "It's just too far for them." So we're doing it in town on Beacon Hill at the Salisbury Club, a neoclassic stone pile that began its life as the home of Nate's great-great-grandparents. Mary and I manage to make it just as cocktails are ending, and Nate does not notice our tardiness. I must say my friend is feeling no pain as he and the rest of us, 150 or so, take our seats. About half the guests are family—the Winsteads came early to New England, prospered, and multiplied—and the rest a mix of North Shore friends and Nate's coworkers from the hospital.

Tonight everyone looks in good form as dessert comes and the toasts (and roasts) to the birthday boy begin. Nate beams and laughs as his siblings and cousins tell "Nate stories." Finally, his turn comes. Nate often stutters, especially when he talks in a group or tells a joke. We are all impressed, therefore, when he asks us to stand and lift our glasses to his mother and father and siblings and Mary, and, stutter-free, asks us to thank them for "all the goodness and happiness in my life. I wouldn't be here without you . . ." Moist-eyed, we cheer and applaud, then sit back down. Soon we are saying our goodbyes. It has been a lovely evening.

Aside from the patrician formality of the setting, which at first nonplussed Nate's work pals, his fiftieth birthday party resembles thousands of others. Or so it seems on the surface—a successful man, a large and happy family, coworkers who have become friends. And it is true: Nate works hard, has an engaging nature, and comes from an extensive and cohesive family. What makes the celebration of his fiftieth extraordinary is that it happened at all, for Nate has Down syndrome. When he was born in the late 1940s, amniocentesis and chromosomal analyses—not to mention legal abortions—did not exist. So Nate could not have been "prevented" the way he could today, the way academic medical leaders like John Knowles recommended during the 1970s.

Instead, like almost everyone else, he entered the world squalling. But then (and now), he could have easily been sidelined into an institution. Indeed, the distinguished neurologists and pediatricians his parents first consulted recommended that they do just that. "Put him in a home," they said. "We know of two excellent private places . . . Your son will be well cared for . . . And you'll have a life." And why should they not? Nate's father was then just back from World War II and studying law at Harvard, and his mother, a champion tennis player and equestrian, was just learning how to cook. They hoped to have a large family. If so, the doctors asked, how could they possibly cope with a "Mongol"? Why didn't they just let Nate go into a "place" and concentrate on having a normal life and other children? "You're such an attractive couple . . . You have everything before you." It seemed everyone was telling them that—certainly the doctors were, including various Winsteads who were then physicians at Harvard and not a few of their more social friends.

Years later, when I asked Nate's mother if she and her husband ever thought of that, of putting Nate in a "place," she said no, it had not occurred to her. "Nate has never been a problem," she said, looking directly at me with her pale blue eyes. "We've had other problems," she continued, not specifying what or who those might be, "but not Nate, not any more than you'd expect of raising any child. He's always been easy." Once she told me that her husband became frustrated with Nate when he was young. Winstead senior is all about action and the world, and with Nate one just has to go a bit slower. Certainly, Nate's father likes bright people and smart talk and accomplishment of all kinds. Anyone who spends time with him can see that. But putting their son in an institution? No, according to his wife, he never even raised the issue. They had servants, for God's sake, he said. They could get Nate all the help he needed right at home and provide extra when he went to school.

Which is what they did. Of course, they sent him to boarding school—a "special one"—when the time came, but then children on each side of the family had gone to boarding schools for generations. Otherwise, Nate lived with them at home and traveled with them on family trips. "He *is* slow, Rob, in some ways," his mother said, "but in others he knows quite a bit. You *know* this— just ask him about the Patriots—he remembers everything! I know he gets frustrated in sports because he's not too coordinated, but *you've* played tennis with him. You can see what he does. And he's probably more normal in a lot of ways than any of the rest of us," she said, chuckling.

It is a late summer afternoon, and Nate's mother and I are sipping daiquiris on her terrace as the others are off somewhere. "The problem with Nate," she says to me as she freshens our drinks, "isn't a problem with Nate, it's a problem with the world." When he was little, she says, strangers made fun of him. Even now, when he lives in Boston on his own during the week, she's sure he faces plenty of "guff" on the streets. But she thinks it does not really get to him much anymore. One of the wisest things she and her family ever did, she says, was early on to heed the advice of an older couple they met who had a child with Down's. "If your son is going to be in the world," she remembers them saying, "then try to arrange his world so it works with him." When he was young, this was not too difficult. Both Nate's parents had deep roots in the area—indeed, his father's people have lived on the same land for over 350 years—and countless cousins lived nearby. Not to mention the benefit of having money. Circumstances could be arranged in Nate's favor.

Of course, they were lucky to find Mary. "You can't overestimate Mary," Nate's mother continues. "We couldn't have done it without Mary. We made sure we paid her well and gave her plenty of time off. I had five other children to look after. I know Mary spent more time with Nate than I did most years. I hope I didn't hurt him in this; I just couldn't do any more than I did."

"And what about Nate's job?" I ask her. "How did he find that?"

"Oh, the *job!*" His mother smiles as we pause for sips. "Isn't it something! Here's Nate, who goes to work every day. My father never worked, at least not like that, and *his* father never worked and Nate's own father *retired* at forty . . . And yet, rain or shine, our son goes in like clockwork. I still time my visits to Bermuda and Florida around Nate's schedule. Can you believe it?" she says, flashing another grin.

When I first knew Nate, the Pilgrim's elevators were manual, and he operated one of them. I expect that the Winsteads somehow arranged the job. But it was up to Nate to keep it, and he did. Several years ago, the Pilgrim's elevators went from manual to automatic, and Nate got switched to sorting packages in the mail room. He doesn't like this work so much. When he was working the elevators, he could greet his North Shore friends—"Hi, Mr. Forbes . . . Mrs. Cabot, nice to see you! How was your trip to Bermuda?" Indeed, sometimes he took them straight to their floors ahead of other visitors, a tendency that his supervisors eventually had to curb. The nice part was that his elevator work kept Nate in contact with people, and its skill requirements were a good fit. He can sort packages all right, but he says it's boring. "No one to talk to, Rob." He wants to change and become a greeter at the hospital's reception area, but he thinks he does not have a chance of getting the job. "I'm too old, Rob. They want the flashy young ones, women. And my supervisor just doesn't like me. It really p-p-p-pisses me off, Rob." I know these frustrations are real for him. I also expect that millions of other older "normal" employees doing simple jobs in complex organizations experience similar ones. Those doing humble work garner little respect these days.

The great sadness of Nate's life, which he mentions sometimes when he's drinking, is that he's stayed single. Not just single, but a New England bachelor in the old sense: only occasional female company. He wanted his life to be otherwise. When he was young, though, people with Down syndrome were discouraged from having a sex life, and marriage then (as now) was mostly out of the question. Add to that the fact that he grew up in a social milieu in which people seldom talked about sex directly. The result, I fear, is that Nate has lived much of his life feeling achingly alone. He has his routines, to be sure: football games in season, which he goes to with a select group of regulars; the newspaper, which he can read a little; and his local bar. Most weekday nights one finds him there, chatting up the female bartenders, knocking back beers and talking sports and politics.

I think of Nate as immensely, if quietly, brave. I have been to watch the football games with him. Once we are near his area, everyone knows him and it's fine. But getting there, or going to the corner grocery with him, is to experience people staring and the occasional snigger. Nate, like other people with Down's I have encountered, smiles at almost everyone with the adoring openness of a five-year-old beaming at his mother. I cannot imagine the hurt he experiences when recipients of his largesse respond with derision. Rare and furtive sex, a narrow path through social gauntlets, and all the frustrations of performing work that is not valued, always and forever: I doubt that I could put up with it.

Not that either lack of sex or de facto prohibition on marriage for those with Down syndrome needs to be. If he is like almost every man with Down syndrome, Nate, if his sperm were tested, would be found to be sterile. Women with Down syndrome may be fertile, and they have a significant chance, on the order of 40 percent, of having a child with Down syndrome, and another 20 percent of their children are either nonviable or have significant problems. But is Down syndrome something that must be prevented as much as possible? Like so much else about the human condition, this depends on the definition of *human* that one adopts. Given how much these definitions vary by tradition and circumstance, should there be some universal criterion? Ironically, when Nate was a young man, John Knowles lived nearby. Though he was not part of the Winstead family's day-to-day social world, they knew him, and Knowles's meadows abutted those of Nate's Winstead cousins. By Knowles's medical logic, though, Nate would not be allowed to live. Indeed, preventing the birth of people with Down syndrome would be normal, and their existence taken as evidence of some parental negligence.

Nate's siblings wonder what will happen to him when their parents die or become incapacitated. His retirement is not too far off. Family thinking runs—and Nate agrees—that he'll probably move full-time back to the North Shore and live in one of the small houses on the family farm. His current weekend routine—a late rise, newspaper sports, lunch at the club, bicycle both ways, beer, TV, family parties—will likely become his daily routine.

The family also thinks, though not as often, about Mary. She does have her sister, but they are not young anymore. Mary must be almost ninety and Alice close to ninety-two. One of these months one of them is going to fall over and have to go into a nursing home—if she survives—and then what will happen to the other? When Mary worked for Nate's family, she lived nearby in a village house the Winsteads owned. Single for life, she moved in with her sister a few years after both retired. Alice has outlived her one child and her husband, and she and Mary have been together for years in Lynn, which is where they started out as sisters in an Irish family with roots in the area. Unlike the Winsteads, however, the family net is thinner. Mary and Alice's nieces and grandnieces and nephews have mostly moved away. So when one of the sisters dies—it does not matter who goes first—the other will soon follow, likely within months. Nate's youngest sister is the one who checks up on them.

I'm wondering about Mary as we drive back to her house in Lynn after Nate's party. Though it's not yet ten o'clock, it has been quite a night for her. So many people came up, and everyone was so nice! She felt embarrassed, she'd forgotten so many names. "I could remember the faces, at least I think I could. Oh, I don't know. We're all getting so damned old." I once asked Mary what she would do with her life if she were young today. "Oh, that's easy," she responded. "I'd be a lawyer. A Boston Irish lawyer, and I bet I would have done very well, thank you."

Like so many of Boston's Irish in the early twentieth century, she was born poor, and, in common with most Irish-American girls of her vintage, did not receive an extensive education. She did not want the convent, she was sure of that, so she went to work for a family, in her case Nate's grandparents and then his parents. They had been good to her, and they saw to it that she had a solid pension and Social Security.

If one looks at Mary's and Nate's lives from the outside in, it is easy to say that they have been disadvantaged ones. However, I expect Mary and Nate would say, though it would be ridiculous to ask them, that they have found their lives to be worth living. Both have crafted circumstances that most of us would find difficult into arrangements that have brought them satisfaction and many occasions for deep pleasure. In doing so, each has moved through the "system" by making few demands on it. Nate's and Mary's temperaments, along with accumulated Winstead determination, wealth, and influence, have permitted them to experience comfortable lives.

THE BULLY IN THE CHINA SHOP

What is it like for others on the margins who go along without benefit of an extensive safety net? With neither private resources nor committed families to back them up, how do they get by? We see them on the streets, and we wonder. In cities large and small, the disparate individuals who live on life's margins these days share at least one feature: they depend on hospitals and their ERs for their medical care. We know this, and we take it for granted. But it was not always so. Indeed, until thirty or so years ago, ERs were not the primary weavers of the medical social safety net. How and why ERs and their hospitals have grown to fill that role is one question. What their dominance means for the vulnerable is another, more poignant one.

I did not drink at Nate's party, for it is a working night. Usually I see emergency patients from 3:00 to 11:00 p.m. two days a week and one weekend a month from 7:00 a.m. to 3:00 p.m., a schedule that best suits my other work without being unfair to ER colleagues. Recently, though, the schedule was tweaked so that I have to work on this Thursday night.

On the way from my parking space to the hospital, I see Chin Lee, one of our frequent ER visitors, walking a little ahead of me toward the bench by the bus stop. Will she be coming in later? I wonder. Usually she does, or she is found and brought in, when it's cold. Tonight it is around fifty degrees Fahrenheit and windy—not cold if you have a decent coat on, but hardly comfortable. I know Chin Lee's age—thirty-seven—because I've seen her medical record. Shuffling in her thin Mandarin-style jacket, pajamas, and paper-thin slippers, her face drawn and gray, she appears much older. About five feet four inches, she likely weighs no more than ninety pounds. None of us in the ER knows how she survives. The nurses frequently give her warm clothes and shoes when she visits, but we never see her wear them on the street. She is a fixture in the neighborhood. Mostly, I see her by the bus stop bench near the Pilgrim and across from Mass Mental, the old state mental hospital that finally shut down in the 1980s. She turns and sees me but gives no sign, which is typical for her.

When Chin Lee comes to the Pilgrim ER on her own, according to her chart, it is usually because she feels sick—she has a fever and cough due to bronchitis or a "walking pneumonia." We treat her, sometimes overnight or for a few days, with antibiotics and food. Sometimes we just give her antibiotic samples we scrounge from the drug company "detail reps" and sequester for patients like her, with no money. When Chin Lee is brought in by others, it is usually because she is raving or incoherent or hypothermic. We warm her up in the ER and consult with the psychiatrists, who give her shots of long-term antipsychotic agents for what they determined years ago was chronic undifferentiated schizophrenia. Sometimes they keep her for observation; sometimes they discharge her to a shelter. Either way, she is soon back on the streets, shuffling quietly in her slippers, a spectral presence on the bus stop bench.

In the old days, before Mass Mental shut down completely, Chin Lee spent much of her daytime life in its neighborhood mental health center, a kind of drop-in place for the chronically afflicted. Before that, she was institutionalized full-time. Is she better off "free"? The state of Massachusetts saved money, to be sure, when, like other states, it began discharging thousands of chronic mentally ill patients from the mid-1960s onward. And it may be that many of them did better with their families or on their own. But for Chin Lee, I wonder. Most states, as well as the federal government, failed to follow up with their promise to establish and fund daytime support centers for those afflicted with mental illness. (One result is that now many of them languish in American prisons, where their psychiatric conditions tend to receive little or no sustained medical attention, according to numerous studies.)

I had just passed Chin Lee, who was perched on the bench, and turned the corner toward the hospital when I heard her yelling, and then a man's voice. What I saw when I turned back was this: Gerald, another of our regular Pilgrim ER visitors, had pushed Chin Lee to the ground and lain down on the bench. She lay whimpering, and he began to curse when he saw and heard me. Gerald may have been a decent person once, but he turned nasty long ago. We, by which I mean all of us who work in the Pilgrim ER, know him well. Physically, he is a bear of a man, florid and puffy on the surface though muscled underneath. In his late forties, he still curses freely, and when confronted, spits, bites, and hits at will.

Chin Lee's medical chart almost fits under one's arm; transporting Gerald's records requires a trolley. This is not because Gerald has any serious ongoing medical problems other than his drinking. It is rather because Gerald likes to sleep in a regular bed and prefers hospital food to what shelters offer. Gerald, who once worked as an ambulance driver, has perfected a simulacrum of a heart attack, a performance he uses to obtain official medical attention. Drunk or sober, and whether sitting in a bar or walking on a sidewalk, when Gerald decides he hankers for hospital food or a bed, he clutches his left chest, screams in pain, and slumps to the ground. On one occasion—it lies buried in one of the early volumes of his chart—his EKG looked slightly off, and Gerald was admitted for a coronary workup. But even then, everything ultimately came back as normal. He does have some risk factors—high cholesterol, heavy use of cigarettes, obesity, family history of coronary artery disease—and he lets everyone know it. He also knows that it can be difficult to establish the diagnosis of heart attack or rule it out by any single test. Tonight I tell him that he had better leave pronto, that I will call the cops on my cell phone if he does not, and that he had better not come back to the bench or show up later in the Pilgrim ER. He swears at me, a bus comes, and he gets on. Chin Lee declines my attention and scrambles for the bench. I go on to the ER.

A few months previously, after a particularly intense spate of Gerald visits, our ER group compiled a year's worth of his Pilgrim performances. The first sentence of his then most recent ER chart said it all: "This is Mr. ———'s 123rd visit to the Pilgrim ER during the past twelve months." Many of those visits ended in overnight hospital stays for evaluation of Gerald's "chest pain." Other than drunkenness, nothing seriously wrong was ever found. The annual cost of this charade, which we asked someone in the billing office to estimate, approached $345,000. Once, a couple of years before, the nurses and social workers persuaded the Pilgrim's legal counsel to petition a court for an order to commit Gerald involuntarily for a one-month stay in an alcohol rehab facility. The judge granted the petition and Gerald went. It turns out that he has both Medicare and Medicaid, so a rehab facility would take him. Hospitals and other inpatient facilities tend to like patients with Medicare *and* Medicaid, for their combined reimbursements approach what can be gleaned from private insurance. Somewhere along the line Gerald gained medicolegal status as disabled due to alcoholism, which is what gave him Medicare and Medicaid as well as a modest monthly stipend. The paradoxical result is that when Gerald came out of rehab, he quickly gained money to resume his usual pursuits. We heard Gerald also availed himself of Boston City (now Boston Medical Center) and Mass General, but we did not verify his visitations there.

If one stands back from the squalid particulars—a large drunken man assaulting a frail woman who talks to herself so he can have a bench to himself—what stands out? Unless one looks carefully, it may be difficult to discern the current roles our hospitals and public policies play. After all, the Pilgrim ER, like others, is open anytime to almost anyone for almost anything remotely "medical." Perhaps nothing is wrong with that. Does not society need at least one health care space where, to paraphrase Robert Frost, when you have to go there, they have to take you in? People like Gerald—bullies who game the system—exist in every sphere, after all. It is unfortunate they get away with it, and some additional measures to restrain the damage they do may be in order, but at first blush it seems that little more could be done.

In fact, more could be done, and at less public cost than is expended currently. Until the late 1970s, many older large U.S. cities, including Boston, maintained dispersed neighborhood-based medical facilities for their residents, not to mention nurses in the public schools and low-cost or no-cost school lunch programs of solid nutritional value. (Boston still maintains a remnant of its community health infrastructure.) People with little money who needed routine or minor care could go to a neighborhood health center, and their civic subsidy was comparatively modest. Moreover, from the implementation of Medicare and Medicaid in the mid-1960s through the mid-1970s, the federal government also funded many additional neighborhood health centers throughout the United States. A similar logic underwrote the 1960s movement for community mental health centers. If people with chronic mental afflictions were able to get their medications and a modicum of therapy in their neighborhoods, the logic ran, they would not destabilize to the point of needing long-term hospitalization.

These structures constitute the endangered ecology of community health approaches. Neighborhood clinics began in earnest early in the last century and gained new life in the 1960s and 1970s. Importantly, assessment studies undertaken during their prime—the late 1960s and early 1970s—suggest that community approaches tended to work better than resource-intensive hospital-based responses. That is, people's health outcomes improved at comparatively modest cost. Indeed, most other economically advanced countries continue with variants of them today, which goes a long way toward explaining why more than twenty other nations have healthier citizens and much lower per capita health care expenditures than we do. So what happened here?

Imagine for a moment that the bus stop bench represents public and private funding for medical care. In the early 1970s, most people had room to sit down. Large hospitals had a place, to be sure (read Gerald before he became so greedy and nasty), but so did neighborhood facilities (read Chin Lee, just out of the inpatient service at Mass Mental). The institutions might not have liked sitting in close proximity, but they managed. But soon the metaphorical Geralds of the institutional world, in the form of the American Hospital Association and others, got tired of sharing the bench and lobbied Congress successfully to reduce seating space for the Chin Lees and expand it for themselves.

Federal funding for modest community-based health infrastructure has not kept up with needs, and cities have not filled in the gap. The primary reason, local leaders say, is that they cannot recover costs from their state government or the feds. For their part, federal and state officials point back to local government even as they reduce funding and tighten eligibility requirements. Neighborhood health centers and day rooms for the mentally afflicted struggle for survival as professional organizations like the American Medical Association and the American Hospital Association, regardless of their rhetoric, mostly stand by and watch. As of 2005, the entire federal budget request for community health centers (not including Medicaid) amounted to $1.79 billion, or approximately 0.07 percent of total American expenditures on health care that year. With that nanocrumb and a few others from the health care cake, 45 million uninsured people are supposed to nourish their need for primary care.

A look around Chin Lee and Gerald's actual bus stop near Longwood Avenue illustrates what happened. During the 1980s, Massachusetts and Boston political leaders as well as the heads of its large teaching hospitals successfully rearranged finance and tax laws so as to encourage hospital expansion of all kinds. Within a few years, new inpatient towers and expansive ambulatory facilities sprawled along the Longwood corridor. Few leaders questioned the actual public need for these kinds of places as compared to the need for other kinds of facilities and providers. But does any city really need five or six major hospital expansions within a mile of each other? Not every large city shares Boston's recent history of hospital boom and semibust, so easily preventable and so freighted with punitive consequence for the vulnerable.

BETRAYAL

A few years have passed. President Bill Clinton has almost finished his speeches about feeling our pain, and George W. has not yet gone national with his compassionate conservatism. Meanwhile, hundreds of formerly "nonprofit" and public hospitals convert to "for-profit" status or sell themselves to Wall Street corporations. Rules for Medicaid eligibility tighten significantly, and millions of workers move from full-time jobs with medical benefits to contract work arrangements that leave them on their own for medical care. I have moved from Boston and the Pilgrim to a Midwestern public university and its Monarch Medical Center.

During a weekday morning between meetings, I walk out of the Monarch's lobby gift shop, candy bar in hand, when I see a clunky old sedan rumble to a stop by the hospital's front door. An older woman pushes open the passenger door and rushes in, screaming for help. She says her husband has just collapsed and points to the car. A large man who looks to be in his sixties is slumped over the wheel, seemingly unresponsive. His breath, which smells like a blend of Juicy Fruit gum and nail polish remover, strongly suggests diabetic ketoacidosis, or DKA. DKA deranges one's metabolism in diverse ways, and, if not controlled, invariably leads to death. When I hurriedly ask his wife about his medical problems, she confirms that her husband is a diabetic and that he has not taken his insulin during the past few days. Without insulin, one's tissues cannot process the sugar in the carbohydrates we ingest. As a result, the body's cells, denied their usual source of energy and ravenous as ever, switch to other mechanisms and start converting fats and proteins into energy. These biochemical reactions produce ketones, a family of molecules that includes acetone, which is common in nail polish remover and why this man's breath smells as it does. The overall process, if carried on long enough, severely disrupts internal fluid balance and acidifies one's blood so that heart and brain no longer work properly and the body effectively shuts down.

We need to get the man out of the car and begin resuscitating him. He barely breathes, no longer responds to my voice or touch, and his pulse is low, around 30. I try mouth to mouth, but that alone will do little. In order to live, this man needs the full gamut—assisted ventilation with oxygen, massive fluids, correction of his blood's acidity and sugar, and emergent attention to his heart, which may be beating slowly because its inherent rhythm has become blocked. Even so, it may be too late. Two hospital employees come out. I ask one to help get the man out of the car and on the ground and the other to call a Code Blue and also alert the ER that we have a man in DKA who is arresting.

A couple of minutes pass, and then an ER crew and their crash cart arrive. And there we are, doing a full-bore Code on a sunny morning on the sidewalk by the entryway. The cardiac monitor indicates that the man's heart has gone into ventricular fibrillation, which means that it is not pumping at all. For the next half hour we do all the appropriate maneuvers, but our efforts are in vain. Since we do not want to pronounce him dead in the parking lot, we move quickly to the ER and try one final round of interventions. Then I let the man's wife, who held his hand in the parking lot and now wails outside the resuscitation room, know that he has "passed." We go down the hall for a quiet place to sit and talk as rivulets of the dead man's saliva dry on the sleeves of my coat.

At some point during the outdoor portion of the Code, I realized I had seen this man before, though I could not remember his name or how we met. When I walked with his wife by the nursing station, it came to me: his name was Cliff, and he delivered and picked up packages for the ER and other departments. "Yes," his widow said. He had been doing it for several years, ever since his earlier employer, a printing company that made envelopes, had cut back. This morning and yesterday, she said, he did not sleep well and got up saying that he didn't feel right. She wanted him to see a doctor, but he was determined to make his delivery rounds first. He just had a few packages. They could go to the hospital (Monarch) and drop them off and then he would think about seeing someone there. Feeling uneasy about him driving on his own, she decided to come along. The packages were still in the backseat, she said. Then she said she needed to call their children and her sister. Did we have a phone? I asked a nurse to sit with her and then left for a luncheon meeting.

Before I left her, though, I asked her about Cliff's insulin. Had he been taking it? No, not in the past four or five days, she answered. Usually he was very careful about his diabetes—checked his blood sugar a couple of times a day at least, paid attention to what he ate, didn't drink. And the insulin? Why had Cliff not taken it? She felt awful about that, she said, sobbing. The package delivery job paid per package delivery, no benefits. Most of the time, they had been able to get by, as she worked part-time for a dry cleaner. But a few months ago Cliff became allergic to his regular insulin, which did not cost that much. His clinic doctor was surprised at the allergy, but she said it happened. The allergy meant he had to switch to a new form of insulin, and that cost a lot. They did not have Medicaid, because they made too much,

and they did not want welfare anyway. But they had trouble sometimes paying for the new version, which cost a multiple of the
old. So Cliff tried to "stretch it." He would take half his dose, or
skip a day.

At the luncheon, which was for department heads and medical
center administrators, the university's chancellor was beaming. A large
man in his early sixties, like Cliff, he proclaimed (I summarize):

> *Today, today is special! Finally, after over two years' work by many
> smart and wonderful people, the governor and a majority of the
> state legislature have agreed to let the Monarch prepare strongly for
> the twenty-first century. We are no longer a public institution, sub-
> ject to the restrictions of state bureaucracy. In two months the
> Monarch will be rechartered as a unique hybrid, a public-private
> partnership with the go-ahead to be as entrepreneurial as we can.
> If things go according to plan, the Monarch, thanks to its newly
> granted authority to issue bonds, will be expanding dramatically in
> certain areas. A state-of-the-art heart center is planned, and a new
> stroke center is in the works.*

We listened and ate our chicken. Still dazed by what had
happened with Cliff before lunch, I was just trying to get through
the meal.

During dessert, the Q&A took place. One of the pediatricians,
a petite Latina who is a true community activist, rose. "Right
now," she said, "we are the hospital of last resort for this state.
Neither this city nor the state has a public hospital. What will
happen to our indigent care? Has the state promised any resources
for them once we go private?" Four months previously, the other
hospital in town that accepted the poor and working poor an-

nounced that it was shutting down in six months, its religious sponsors tired of the deficits. What would their and our patients do come summer? Would we be seeing all of them in the Monarch ER—which would probably become nightmarishly busy? And what about follow-up in the clinics? Had not the chancellor said earlier that new financial rules would be coming into play for the clinics and what he termed "elective care"? He answered that the old state subsidy for indigent care, some $15 million per year, was being phased out.

I came home that evening angry and disgusted. Part of my work then included service as the medical center's "chief ethics officer." It was not a job I had been recruited for or sought, but a duty the chancellor added on to help the hospital recover from a previous ethics scandal. They—the Monarch's administration—needed to demonstrate to the state legislature that they had beefed up oversight mechanisms to prevent serious future transgressions in patient care. It turned out, however, that the post came with no administrative mechanisms or resources to give the chief ethics officer any clout. I had accepted it because the chancellor had asked me—I was new to the place—and because in return the medical center had agreed to hire an assertive lawyer-ethicist to head its institutional review board (IRB), which I thought needed some rigor.

Even so, I had no illusions that our leaders truly wanted organizational ethics introduced into the center's daily life. Beginning in the mid-1990s, medical and hospital leaders, not to mention corporate CEOs, began regularly talking up "integrity," "ethics," and "professionalism" as central to their enterprises. When it comes to the day-to-day grind of calculating institutional and personal advantage, however, few leaders want an ethicist examining their administration's moral books. If they did, they would include one to opine on large-scale change, just as they do a score of lawyers. But that rarely happens. Except for IRBs and the occasional ceremony, ethicists tend to be kept out of the inner circles. One result is that they tend not to know what *really* goes on, and when they find out, they tend to be sidelined from the process of adjusting the fundamentals. Meanwhile, a stripped-down expediency drives the big decisions.

Unless something goes seriously wrong—or rather, unless something serious goes wrong that the public might find out about—an ethicist's actual functions tend to the ornamental and cosmetic. During the two years I held the post of chief ethics officer, which the Monarch, incidentally, quietly retired as it went from public to private, I lived with the expectation that if something from the organization's murk should bubble into public view, I would at best be charged with cleaning it up, at worst be the designated fall guy. Either way, I probably would not know about it in advance of or during a crisis unless the administration got wind that the media sensed a potential scandal.

What fueled my anger that evening was my sense of how this new public-private model would likely play out for people like Cliff. The Monarch's switch and the impending collapse of the other hospital might spell the end of all but emergency interventions for the uninsured. A lack of regular care for the needy could extend from the city to the eastern portion of the state. I felt disgusted that I was a part of the operation, periodically put on a podium to provide a moral imprimatur for biomedical moves that, taken as a whole, betrayed the common good in favor of narrow interests.

If one were to characterize in a word our medical system as

compared to Canada's or France's, one might call ours "private" and theirs "public" or "socialized." And up to a point, one would be correct. Although France, like other Western European countries, permits private medical practice and hospitals, and Canada, until recently, did not, the comparative surprise may be this: in America, which we think of as the realm of "private" medical care, approximately 50 percent of our total expenditures on health care come from the public purse. Moreover, our public half is as large in percentage of gross economic output and larger in per capita expenditure than what citizens of *any* country spend, public and private combined, on their health care. Yet in terms of commonly employed health criteria—rates of infant mortality, average life expectancy, "quality-adjusted life years," and so forth—U.S. rates lie at or near the bottom in comparison with economically advanced countries and on a par with some developing nations, such as Costa Rica.

Given our resources and all that we know about disease prevention, the value of adequate nutrition for children, and effective tactics for managing common chronic illnesses, can any approach be less intelligent than ours? In today's America, when we say we embrace being *human* and *humane*, what do we mean?

8

As Night Draws Nigh

From birth to death, each of us lives both alone and with others. Along the way, our attachments to a few people—parents, partners, children, close friends—give our lives considerable meaning. Yet when it comes to dying in America these days, many of us depart the world, if not entirely alone, then in the company of mere strangers, the ones like me who staff hospitals. Meanwhile, those who have mattered most to us remain just offstage, in an ICU lounge perhaps, waiting for a nurse's announcement that we have "passed." Have you been with someone who is dying? At the moment when someone close to us may be most alone—the minutes and hours when death is approaching—it seems the merest decency to stay with that person if we are able and circumstances permit (unless the dying person can still decide for himself and insists otherwise). What does it feel like to be close to someone one cares for who is dying? To be sure, the memory remains—hauntingly, probably, at least for a time—but it should not supplant earlier memories. Instead, it is likely to enhance one's sense of having shared a life. What else do we have?

When death finally looms, as it inevitably does, we practitioners of "health science," who tend to shy away from even mention of dying, belittle one of the primary roles of ancient healers (and priests). Instead of being with the dying, of serving our patients and their families as death's familiar, its knowing witness, all too often we retract our necks into our white coats like turtles, mumble in technospeak, and step backward, slowly.

Like others providing critical care, I have been with many dying people. Just as I have also been with many who seemed to be dying—who were, in fact, clinically dead, at least for moments—before our interventions revived them. Until my father died in 2004, however, I had not been at the side of a dying family member. Because I have a medical license and know something of the terrain of dying in hospital, I was able to help my father experience a more comfortable death. But one does not have to be medically credentialed to be able to help a loved one during the final hours and days. Unlike Mike Murphy, my father did not die of cancer. If he had, then we, his family and he, would have known more or less when he was to die. Although advanced cancers may cause immense suffering as they kill, most of them signal their endgame well in advance. Which means that the afflicted, or at least his or her physicians, may exercise considerable agency in shaping his final time, as Mike did. Indeed, the hospice movement began as a means to help people with terminal cancer experience their final months with a modicum of comfort and dignity. That we who practice medicine in America do not let most of our cancer patients know they are dying until their time is quite short—

from a few days to a couple of weeks—does not do us credit. Instead of acknowledging the truth, which our patients may sense but are unable to confirm without us, we all too often confuse them right up to the end with unrelenting and burdensome treatment. Only when death appears imminent do we tell them they are dying and suggest hospice and palliative care.

Most people in their seventies and older, however, do not die of cancer. Like my father, who died just before his eighty-sixth birthday, they tend to die of less predictable processes. Current knowledge concerning when someone with heart disease, serious lung problems, diabetes, a degenerative neurological condition, or one of their attendant infections—the leading noncancer causes of death among those over sixty-five—will die is not nearly as precise or accurate as our knowledge of when metastatic cancer has gained the final upper hand. Indeed, we physicians are not even good at predicting the short-term outcome of most acute hospitalizations for people in these situations.

What does the medical profession's present ignorance mean for you or for someone you care for? Not knowing with much reliability when one will die means that until the very end—when death stares at us point-blank—doctors have little idea when our aggressive treatments become futile. We may know the five-year survival curves for groups with severe congestive heart failure, advanced renal disease, and Alzheimer's, but we don't know whether this or that episode of pneumonia or renal failure will end someone's life until it almost has. Again, this is not true for advanced cancers, but it is for almost everything else. In hindsight we doctors may be able to see that someone's death was imminent, but our foresight remains myopic. This is one reason—in my view the major one—why older people dying of heart and lung disease, chronic neurological afflictions, kidney disease, and the infections that often complicate all of them die by an overwhelming margin in hospitals, not hospices or homes, and then often in ICUs.

Even so, experience persuades me that there are better and worse ways to die in a hospital. My father, thanks to a variety of circumstances, died in a better way. Though possessed of an adventuresome streak—he contemplated overnight sailing trips up into his mid-seventies—my father took pride in approaching life as an engineer, which is how he was trained. The accurate definition of a situation and methodical attention to the details of its possible outcomes characterized his approach to work and life. He did not believe in God or an afterlife. Skeptical of what could happen in complex settings like hospitals, he thought advance directives, in the form of a living will and durable power of attorney for health care, were prudent, and he made sure his doctors, wife, children, attorney, and the local hospital each had copies. He gave Jean, his wife of twenty-five years and my stepmother, legal power to make decisions when he could not.

Fortunately for him, until his late seventies Dad's health had not presented many problems. But then he started to experience difficulty breathing. It turned out that the lining of his lungs had thickened so much that oxygen could no longer pass easily from the atmosphere into his blood. The condition is called interstitial fibrosis. None of his pulmonary experts could figure out why this had occurred, which is not unusual for the condition. Living in the Rockies did not help, but my father and Jean decided not to move to a lower altitude. Instead, he adapted, and a portable oxygen canister entered the picture. Though he slowed down physically and mentally and gave up much of his civic committee work, Dad continued to write letters to the editor and agitate by phone for various town projects until just before his final illness. Indeed, I think Dad's final illness may have surprised him and Jean—it came on so fast. I know it caught my brother Bill, who lives in Northern California, unawares, just as it did my stepsister Linda, who lives near Dad and Jean, my stepbrother Jeff, who lives in New York City, and me, living in New Orleans at the time.

I wrote the following account a few days after my father died. I chose to write it plainly, sensing that I would want to explore other dimensions later. Coincidentally, my mother, his former wife of thirty-four years, was also ill at the time, though she survived. Although I had not imagined writing this book at the time I wrote about my father's death, I reproduce the account here to illustrate how a "better death" can unfold.

January 16, 2004

Four days ago my brother Bill called from Santa Cruz, California, to tell me in New Orleans that our mother was entering the hospital in Santa Cruz with pneumonia. Three weeks previously I had come from New Orleans to see her at Christmas, when she was ill with what seemed to be bronchitis. At that time my brother, who lives near her, and I encouraged her to see her doctor, but she refused. She thought she would get better on her own. She feared going into the hospital. "Everyone I know gets sick there," she said, not without reason. She is eighty-four and lives independently. She still works occasionally, in fact, selling antiques. Finally, though, she went, after my brother took her to the ER and the ER doctor insisted she stay. He was confident she would get better. When I heard the news, I was on my way to a medical conference in the Northeast. My brother said there was no need to come to California to see Mom; he would keep me informed.

As a young man, my brother Bill raced cars and motorcycles; now he restores vintage Ferrari engines. We get along fine.

Late the next day Linda, my stepsister, called from western Colorado to say that Marty, my father, had been taken to the hospital Friday night with breathing trouble. Pneumonia was the hospital diagnosis, but with the twist of low blood pressure and low oxygen content in the blood. Jean, his wife, had called the paramedics when he seemed barely responsive. They gave him high-flow oxygen by face mask and took him to the ER, where the staff put him on dopamine, a medicine to stabilize his blood pressure, and moved him to the ICU. His heart was beating slowly and then fast with runs of ventricular tachycardia. Not a good sign in an old man—my father is almost eighty-six—with a history of fibrosis in his lungs. Though his heart had always been strong, I thought my father had likely experienced a heart attack, but Linda said the ER physician said the EKG did not show it.

Sunday morning I talked with the ICU physician. Dad was alert, oriented, and breathing easily with the help of high-flow oxygen. He had eaten a little and was talking to Jean. The chemical tests, though, confirmed a myocardial infarction—heart attack— and according to a portable echocardiogram, his heart's pumping chamber, the left ventricle, was not doing well. His ejection fraction, which measures the ability of the left ventricle to empty itself, was only 35 percent. His physician and I puzzled about this. With an ejection fraction so low, he should be in florid heart failure, but he was not. No swelling of the legs, no deterioration of kidney function. Stable blood chemistries except for the cardiac muscle enzymes.

Either the echo test was off—it was a portable, after all, and sub-ject to considerable variation—or it was accurate and he would get worse.

He got worse. Sunday night Linda called to say that his breath-ing was rapid and that he had been hallucinating. I had better come. Dad's doctor, whom I spoke with shortly after, seconded Linda. I also talked with Jean, who sounded levelheaded but tired. She had stayed with him in the ICU Saturday night and not slept well. I called my brother and told him we needed to go to Colorado.

Bill and I met at the Denver airport early the next evening to catch the same flight over the Rockies to western Colorado. Bad weather canceled that flight, though, so we rented a car and my brother drove us west. Mom was getting better, he said; she should be fine. She sounded better on the phone when I talked with her on Sunday, I said. Our parents had divorced over twenty-five years ago and had barely spoken since. Ironic, we said, that they each en-tered a hospital on the same day with the same diagnosis. Quick smiles. We were amused at the coincidence but doubted they would be. Too many hard feelings between them still.

We got to the hospital in Glenwood Springs around midnight. It was clear and cold. Linda met us at the door of the ICU. Dad, whom everyone calls Marty, was not doing well. Jean lay beside him in his bed, touching his shoulder and face. Dad was breathing rapidly; the oxygen was on maximum flow. He appeared to be dozing. The bedside monitor displayed a rapid and regular heart rate, adequate blood pressure, and lowish oxygen saturation—88 per-cent. (An oxygen saturation of 88 percent when someone is on high-flow inhaled oxygen means that their lungs are able to extract only about 60 percent of what normal lungs do on room air.) Jean said he had been asking for us. We touched his shoulders and arms and talked to him, and he recognized us and knew where he was. The nurse—K.C.—came in and out to moisten his lips and tried to make him comfortable. Linda wet a towel and put it on his forehead. Telling him what I was doing, I felt his legs and the top of his feet—warm, no significant edema, and lively pedal pulses. But he did not look long for this world. I was used to all this; my brother was not, however, and he looked shocked. He had not seen Dad in a few years; I had visited last August.

I excused myself and went to the nursing station to talk with the nurses and check his chart. For a moment I thought the nurses and I might have a difficult time with each other. They knew I was a professor at Tulane Medical School, as Jean had told them. But when I asked to see the chart, they refused. But wait a moment, I said. They responded that they could not, that the new federal patient confidentiality regulations—HIPAA—required written patient consent. Which meant I had to go to medical records the next morning to get the form, the nurse said. Then, if my father agreed and signed the form, I could see his chart. Really? I could call his doctor if I wished. But then the nurses told me his story and his test results and we began to establish a rapport. They did not like the rigidity of the new regulations either. I decided to wait until morning to call his doctor, who would be in around seven anyway.

The lab tests confirmed the heart attack, but they also showed something else. The lung infection—a streptococcus—had spread to the blood. Dad was septic, which is bad in anyone but often devastating in the elderly and even in younger patients with other serious co-conditions.

My father had been clear that he did not want aggressive medical care if he was at the end of his life. Everyone knew this and accepted it, and his living will left no doubt. He had been DNR—do not resuscitate—from the start, which is why the ICU staff did not place him on a ventilator. Antibiotics and supplemental oxygen are not extraordinary measures, however, at least by most standards, including mine. Would he make it with just those treatments and perhaps a couple of others for comfort? Morphine, in addition to being an excellent medicine for pain, does two things that can help people with acute lung failure: it dilates the pulmonary vessels, thereby increasing blood flow, and reportedly it cuts one's sensation of not getting enough air—"air hunger," we call it. But at some point in the past Dad had experienced an episode in which his blood pressure bottomed out after a morphine dose. And so he was on mild doses of Demerol, which is acceptable for pain, but not known to help air hunger or pulmonary blood flow. Demerol can also lead to unpleasant hallucinations, and I do not like to use it.

Years ago when I was a medical student doing my ICU rota-tion, my first patient was a big man in his mid-eighties with pneu-monia who had become septic. Active and well before his illness, he, too, had made himself DNR. For the first few days his conscious-ness was clouded, and we feared the worst. I spent a lot of time with him day and night, as did the nurses and ICU resident. He recovered fully, and when he did so we talked about his great love, which was chamber music. He talked about cellos and Bach and music festivals and then went home. Memories of this came back as I was listening to the ICU nurses in Colorado tell me about Dad.

Jean asked Dad if he was thirsty—"Yes"—and the nurse brought in a cup of water and a straw. He sipped a little. "Do you hurt?" Jean asked. "No," he responded. "Bill and Rob drove from Denver," she told him again. "Good," he said; "I know." Almost in turn, Bill, Linda, and I would get choked up and turn away for a moment before turning back. After a little more of this I motioned to Jean and Bill and Linda to go in the other room and told Dad that we would be right back. Ever so slightly, he nodded. We assembled in an adjacent room.

Even when someone may seem out of it or perhaps in a coma, around the very sick it is important to always talk with them and not about them. When the four of us had been in with Dad, I could see from my relatives' gestures and body language that my family wanted my medical opinion, that they were on the verge of questioning me and I on the verge of responding. That's why I motioned us aside.

Dad is dying. I know this, and I think Jean, who spent last night with him, and Linda probably know this too. But they, like Dad, are exhausted, and Bill is in shock. He has not seen Dad for several years. In the side room, I sensed that Jean, Linda, and Bill wanted an answer. Was Dad at the absolute end? Should we let him go? "What do you think?" is what one of them asked, I cannot remember which one.

Though tired, I felt present, and I was not sure how to answer. Time flows one way in life, and I did not want to participate in ending my father's until I was sure he had no chance of recovery and that more time for him only meant more agony. I thought I did not yet know all the details. How long had he been on the antibiotic, for instance? In medical school the big man with pneumonia who had become septic at one point looked like a goner too, but he had recovered. To give my father a modest dose of morphine would probably ease his hunger for air, especially if we added a small dose of a sedative, such as Ativan. But the drugs would likely bottom out his blood pressure, in which case he would fade out. His agony would end and so would his life. I wanted to wait and talk with his doctor first thing in the morning. I said also that all of us were very tired—Jean had not slept the previous night, for instance, when she stayed with my father. For the moment, Dad was holding his own; his vital signs had been stable for several hours. We all needed some rest before we said our goodbyes. I could not tell from their reactions what Jean, Linda, and Bill thought of my opinion, but they accepted it. Jean, Bill, and I drove home to Dad and Jean's, and Linda returned to her place. K.C., the nurse, would call my cell phone if Dad's condition worsened. Otherwise we would be back by seven, when his doctor usually arrived. It was around 1:30 in the morning.

Four hours later K.C. called to say that Dad was getting worse: his sats (a measure of oxygen in the blood) were falling, his breathing was more rapid and labored. I got up, took a shower, and put on a sport jacket. I wanted to be nicely dressed for my father. Then I awakened my brother and Jean, and she called Linda. We met around an hour later in the ICU. Despite full supplemental oxygen, Dad looked desperate for air. His blood pressure was adequate, but his heart rate was up and his sats were down in the mid-eighties, which meant his blood's hemoglobin was probably carrying only about half the ideal amount of oxygen. I reached his doctor by telephone and described the situation, and she agreed it was time, as did K.C.

Then I shared our thoughts with my family. If we gave Dad a little morphine and Ativan, I said, he would become more comfortable and we could each say our goodbyes. They agreed. K.C. and I placed ourselves on either side of Dad's bed and I told him that we were going to give him medicine to help his breathing. I said to him that he would not have to struggle anymore. K.C. gave him the drugs by IV. In a few minutes his posture and breathing eased. I told him that his time on earth was coming to an end and that I loved him. I touched him with a recent photograph of my children. Then I took the oxygen tubes off him, kissed his forehead, and wished him peace. The last words I heard from him were "Thank you." Then I excused myself and Bill, Linda, and Jean each had time with him. Afterward, they said he knew they were there. Then the four of us together stood by the bed, touched him, and watched him die.

The final dying took about five minutes. He would seem dead—no respirations, no pulse, no blood pressure—and then he would make a single gasp for air, a reflex action coming from his lower brain as his upper brain gave out. It is very hard to watch someone go through this. One wants to reach out and either bring them back or do something to stop it. I had seen this many times before, so it was not so hard for me even though it was my father. But it must have been awful for Bill, Jean, and Linda. Even so, I think it was better for all of us, including Dad, to have this experience than its alternative, which would have been to administer high doses of morphine and Ativan in quick succession. That I would not do, if only because I would have thought of myself forever after as someone who killed his father, not helped him. If my relatives are angry at me for putting them through those unbearable final minutes—Dad was comfortable, I am sure—I hope they forgive me. I went with the comfort doses for another reason, too. According to Jean, Dad when well insisted that she promise she would not arrange a funeral or public memorial service for him but instead just simple cremation and pour his ashes into the Colorado River, which flowed near their house. Since honoring his wishes meant that we, his survivors, would forgo any formal acknowledgment of his life and passing, I thought that letting him go over a few minutes as opposed to a minute, even though it was difficult to witness, let us die a little *with him the way one does at the funeral or memorial service of a loved one. In any case, I served him as well as I know how.*

Had I been alone in the room with my newly dead father, I would have stayed for a time—a half hour perhaps—and gazed at his face and head. I have done this with a few patients I have known personally. Their features seem to settle in and become taut at the same time, like a death mask by Houdon, the Enlightenment sculptor. One thinks one sees something new and essential about the person, but what that is, I cannot say. As it was, I gazed at my dead father for a few minutes before we all left. He looked noble.

We were hungry, and we decided to eat out before going home to Dad and Jean's. I joked that I wanted a Bloody Mary, which I really did, but the only open restaurant did not serve alcohol. Each of us ate a large breakfast and talked, but I cannot remember what was said. Then we went to Jean and Dad's. Later that afternoon, after Jeff arrived from New York, we read my father's will. The next morning my brother and I drove to Denver and flew back to our respective homes.

ALTERNATIVE SCENARIOS

Most medical deaths of the elderly (as compared to, say, young people dying from trauma) have a few key moments when the duration of the dying process hangs on a single decision. My father's situation was typical of this in that his dying could have been prolonged had a few details or choices been different. When the paramedics arrived, suppose my father had had a pulse and blood pressure but had been unresponsive and not breathing (as opposed to how he was, minimally responsive and minimally breathing).

Whether or not Jean told them of his DNR status, the paramedics would likely have put in an artificial airway—an endotracheal tube—and begun ventilating him. They would have done so because he possessed vital signs—a pulse and blood pressure—and emergency field protocols specify ventilatory support when they are present, regardless of the circumstances. This makes intuitive sense: in emergent moments, one does not know why a patient stops breathing, but one does know how to maintain that patient's breathing function by other means. And if one does not intervene right then, the person dies. No one, I venture, wants paramedics to hold back life-extending treatments in such situations.

If Dad had arrived in the Glenwood Springs ER with a breathing tube in place, the emergency staff would have placed him on a ventilator before admitting him to the ICU. As it was, he arrived barely breathing. When elderly patients arrive with compromised breathing and signs of shock—low blood pressure and pulse—often ER staffs intubate their airways and do other measures to support their vital functions. I suspect the only reason the ER staff did not intubate my father was that Jean arrived with his DNR documents, which explicitly stated that he did not want to be on a ventilator. Dad had been dealing with his pulmonary fibrosis for seven or eight years, and he expected it would eventually kill him. He anticipated that if his lungs failed, artificial ventilation would not help them back to baseline but just prolong the inevitable, an opinion his physicians and I shared. My father's prescience about the dubious value of ventilators for his situation turned out to be crucial. Had he gone on a ventilator, he might have continued "living" for weeks in the Glenwood ICU as his heart and lungs, and then his kidneys and liver, finally gave out. During this time he would not have been fully awake—sedatives required to make him tolerate a tube in his trachea would ensure that—and tubes would have been in his veins and urethra as needles frequently punctured his skin. For what purpose?

Can we generalize from my father's experience? Two things stand out, one medical and one administrative. For elderly patients experiencing a rapid decline in lung function in the context of widespread bodily failure, a key medical decision concerns whether to go on a ventilator or not. Early proponents of ventilators and ICUs, such as Henry Beecher, the influential Harvard anesthesiologist mentioned in Chapter 6, saw them as *bridging* technologies to carry patients over crises that would otherwise prove lethal. They did not envision them as standard interventions for elderly people suffering multiple organ system failures at the end of life. But that is often how ventilators are deployed today. Furthermore, the reality is that once such patients go on a ventilator, usually considerable time passes before they are taken off or die so encumbered.

The euphemistic skew of standard hospital rhetoric does not help patients and families in these situations. Instead of discussing the dubious value of continuing artificial ventilation for Grandma or Grandpa's unstoppable decline, we talk instead about taking them off "life support" or withdrawing "life-sustaining" measures. Indeed, we insist they sign documents that say no more "life support." *Artificial ventilation* and *life support*, however, do not resonate as existential equivalents. Sometimes, to cover the slippage, we doctors try to finesse the issue. We may recommend a brief trial of "life support"—say three days on a ventilator—in such situations, which may be deemed acceptable. One should be aware, however, that often the three days drag on to a couple of weeks. Some ethicists maintain that stopping artificial ventilation of a patient unable to breath on her own after a trial period on the ventilator is morally neutral. In real life, though, family members struggle with "pulling the plug." They feel, many have told me, as if they are "killing" their loved one. Which is one reason the plug typically does not get pulled until weeks have passed

What kept my father from a ventilator-extended dying process was not just his completion in advance of a living will with DNR clauses and a durable power of attorney in favor of Jean, but the fact that she had the documents with her when Dad arrived in the ER. As a backup, he previously had sent copies to the hospital's medical records office, where he knew someone, as well as to his physicians. Had Jean not had the documents with her in the ER, however, it is likely that Dad would have gone on a ventilator for at least a few days until his local physician and the hospital and Jean had sorted out the paperwork.

COMFORT MEASURES

When I first showed the account of my father's death to a literary colleague, she said that what "jumped off the page" were the words that I chose smaller doses so that I would not remember myself "as someone who had killed his father, not helped him." Can one make a valid moral distinction between "comfort measures," such as the small doses of morphine and the sedative Ativan we administered my father for air hunger, and larger doses of the same drugs that would have provided comfort but also hastened his death?

"Yes" is the response of the Western moral philosophy that forms the intellectual backbone of bioethics. When artificial means of extending the dying process, such as ventilators and ICUs, first became regular features of hospital landscapes in the 1960s and 1970s, medical leaders called upon early bioethicists to devise ethical frameworks for physician behavior toward those experiencing the extended dying common in these new settings. Perhaps because many early bioethicists were trained in moral philosophy and religious studies, mainly at Catholic universities, they responded by refurbishing a venerable philosophical notion: the principle of double effect, first put into words by Thomas Aquinas, the thirteenth-century Christian theologian and philosopher.

In his *Summa Theologica* (Part II-II, Question 64, Article 7), Aquinas maintains that "nothing hinders one act from having two effects, only one of which is intended, while the other is beside the intention." The context here, however, is not medical, but rather that of self-defense. If a person is attacked, self-defense may have two effects, he notes: "one, the saving of one's life; the other, the slaying of the aggressor." The justification of self-defense rests on characterizing the defensive action as a means to a justified goal—self-preservation. Aquinas then adds the constraint that "though proceeding from a good intention, an act may be rendered unlawful if it be out of proportion to the end." In other words, moderation or proportionality is required, even in repelling someone attempting to slay you.

Over seven hundred years have passed since Aquinas's death, and hundreds of theologians and philosophers have written about his principle of double effect, which now exists in many versions. In a medical context, the principle is directed at well-intentioned agents who question whether they may cause a potential harm in order to bring about a good end. Of overriding moral importance is the stipulation that it be impossible to bring about the good end without also causing the harm. Most versions assume that four conditions must be present:

1. The contemplated action in itself must be good or at least indifferent.
2. One intends the good effect and not the bad effect.
3. The good effect must not be produced by means of the bad effect.
4. The good effect must be sufficiently worthwhile to compensate for allowing the bad effect.

As one might imagine, each of these conditions generates controversy, with the most heated occurring around the subjectivity of intention. For example, when the likely outcome of an intervention—say, death from administration of very large doses of narcotics to a dying patient in severe pain from cancer—is readily foreseeable, how can an observer reliably discern that the agent did not intend the "bad" effect—hastened death—but only the "good"—relief of severe and ultimately unnecessary pain? Even so, medical statutes in all fifty states that regulate physician behavior around the dying permit physicians to act according to the principle of double effect, and many make explicit reference to it.

No state except Oregon, however, explicitly permits physicians to assist patients who want their doctors to make them dead.

EUTHANASIA IN FACT, IF NOT IN NAME

Putting aside Oregon, the ground rules for dying *pace* double effect are nevertheless hardly clear. As the physician Timothy Quill eloquently noted in 1997, before Oregon passed its law, the conceptual murkiness of double effect tends to inhibit open end-of-life communication between physicians, patients, and their families:

> *Double effect, by relying on the fiction that the clearly foreseeable consequences of an act are not intended, often permits doctors deliberately to cause death, but because the provision of drugs for the same purpose remains criminal in all circumstances, the law prevents open consultation with the patient, the family and other physicians.*

In short, "justification by double effect . . . may function as a 'fig leaf' for euthanasia," as some physicians have maintained. For the chronically ill who are close to dying or in its early stages, such "fig leaves" approach the bizarre. New York State regulations, for example, permit euthanasia of a sort, though they never call it that. If you are approaching death in New York and find your situation intolerable, your physician may legally fulfill your request to be placed in a medically induced coma without hydration and nutrition until you die. Such "terminal sedation" can take a while—from days to two weeks—which may mean that you spend your final time experiencing pain—sedatives do not relieve that—but unable to express yourself as you dehydrate and starve while your family, grimly, maintains a vigil. Is this death with dignity?

ORDINARY AND EXTRAORDINARY

Suppose you have become *very* old and your senses and much of your mind have ceased to work. No longer able to live independently, you now live in a nursing home or, less commonly, at home with extensive care from paid strangers. You have experienced a stroke or two, occasional pneumonia and other infections, as of your urinary tract, and you can no longer feed or provide any other care for yourself. You are utterly dependent on others. What should you or your family do when the next infection or neurological degradation occurs? There is no easy answer. But American law, as determined by state and federal courts over the past three decades, is clear about what is legally permitted. A seriously ill or dying person is not required to accept treatments, including food and water by artificial means, such as a feeding tube. This may sound straightforward on paper, but in everyday life complications often intrude. The most common, I venture, is that the person in her late eighties or nineties did not, when possessing decisional capacity, give clear instructions. Because she did not, the onus typically falls on the family. Even when the dying person has made his wishes known, the family does not always agree, however.

My grandmother, Anna Sommer, died during her ninety-ninth year in a nursing home. Although she had become a widow in her late seventies, she continued living in her family home until her early nineties, when independent life became too difficult for her. When she moved to a nursing home, Grandma still possessed mental agility, and she and her three children—two daughters and a son—agreed that she and they did not want what they viewed as "extraordinary" interventions if her underlying condition verged on the vegetative. When it finally did—strokes made her more or less immobile during her ninety-sixth year, and she was already blind and quite hard of hearing—it seemed at first that the family agreed on a proper course for future care: comfort care, nothing "extraordinary," which they defined as DNR, no antibiotics for systemic infections, and no artificial hydration or nutrition.

Grandma's eldest, a daughter, always lived near her mother and saw her more or less daily. But my mother and uncle lived far away from their mother and saw her only a few times a year. Although the three siblings tended to agree when they met around their mother's bedside in response to one of her medical crises, my aunt, the child who actually spent time with her on a daily basis, found she could not stick with the agreements when her mother experienced another setback and she was alone with her. When Grandma developed a serious systemic infection, for example, my aunt overcame her hesitation to "do nothing," as she put it, and instead agreed to treatments with intravenous antibiotics, nutrition, and hydration. Then my uncle and mother would arrive, and the three would agree not to authorize the next step, a feeding tube. But when the younger two departed and my aunt remained, she later said she felt morally compelled to approve the feeding tube. To do otherwise, she said, felt like abandoning her mother, or worse. Eventually, Grandma died of an overwhelming infection, approximately two years after she first underwent placement of a feeding tube.

Some religious traditions make significant distinctions between "ordinary" and "extraordinary" medical interventions and some do not. Both my grandparents regularly attended Lutheran services, but my mother and her siblings do so uncommonly or not at all. In any case, my understanding is that none of them queried Lutheran doctrine to find direction for their end-of-life planning. In comparison, I have cared for many Catholic patients and families who actively sought guidance from their confessors. The late Pope John Paul II could not have been clearer on the Roman Catholic definition of "basic health care" and the obligation to provide it to anyone alive, including someone in a "vegetative state." As John Paul II declared in 1994 to a congress on "life-sustaining treatments": "I should like particularly to underline how the administration of water and food, even when provided by artificial means, always represents a *natural means* of preserving life, not a medical act. Its use, furthermore, should be considered, in principle, *ordinary*" (emphasis in original).

LIVING FOR OTHERS

Around the dying, as around the chronically ill or incapacitated, we like to think that families come together, and many do. But many, like Betsy's in Chapter 3, also come apart. Along with fracturing a sick person's body, serious illnesses may fracture a person's family, especially when more than one generation is involved or the family is a blend of step-relations and half-siblings. In most families of dying patients, everyone involved will likely engrave on their memories how each behaved to the dying and each other. Emotions almost invariably run raw, especially if the dying extends in time or awfulness. Even witnessing a "better death" of someone we love strips us to the bone. If one or another family member leaves the experience feeling profoundly betrayed by a relative, by the hospital, by a physician or nurse, or even by their lesser self, they may never get over their anger. As I hope the narrative of my father's death demonstrates, there is one essential requirement for being close with a dying person: the letting go of self-concern. This may include past hurts one has experienced at the dying person's hands (or those of one's assembled relatives). Maintaining mindful compassion may be difficult. Authentic caring for a dying person, however, calls on us to imagine and respond to the other in all his or her fullness, even as that life runs out before ours.

Notes and Sources

Preface

xii   *Compared to those in other countries, older Americans dying in hospitals:* On what happens with dying patients in hospitals, anthropologist Sharon R. Kaufman provides many sobering examples in her *. . . And a Time to Die: How American Hospitals Shape the End of Life* (New York: Scribner, 2005). In her recent book *Final Exam: A Surgeon's Reflections on Mortality* (New York: Knopf, 2007), Pauline W. Chen gives a personal account of the inadequate training physicians receive for treating patients experiencing the final stages of chronic illness.

xiii   *In these pages, therefore, I have tried to write:* The phrase *biomedical-industrial complex* echoes President Eisenhower's memorable "military-industrial complex" of his 1961 farewell address. Eisenhower did not question that "our arms must be mighty." What concerned him was the "acquisition of unwarranted influence, whether sought or unsought," by such a complex over the "very structure of our society." Its "total influence—economic, political, even spiritual," he warned, could cause us to lose our "balance." Transposing the concept into the world of health and disease, I share his concerns and goal, the preservation of balance at the individual and social levels.

        A key event in the development of the biomedical-industrial complex was Congressional passage of the Bayh-Dole Act (Public Law 96-517) in 1980. The law's primary intent was to encourage growth of tech-based small businesses by permitting them at no cost to own patents that arose from federally sponsored research. Universities successfully lobbied to be included as "small entities" with the understanding that they would not develop the patented technologies but instead license the patents. Academic-industrial partnerships took off in the late 1980s with the passage of the Technology Transfer Act of 1986. These two pieces of legislation encouraged universities such as MIT and Stanford, who were concerned about the fall-off in Defense Department research contracts as the cold war faded, to ramp up their technology transfer operations.

In brief, the post-1980s system operates as follows: public funds from the National Institutes of Health and the National Science Foundation provide universities with research infrastructure at little cost to themselves, corporations get the research for free or close to it, and both benefit from commercial applications of that research. Some physicians, such as Thomas Stossel at Harvard, vigorously support the arrangement. See his editorial, "Regulating Academic-Industrial Research Relationships—Solving Problems or Stifling Progress?," *New England Journal of Medicine* 353, no. 10 (2005): 1060–65. Many knowledgeable observers, however, express caution, such as Derek C. Bok, *Universities in the Marketplace: The Commercialization of Higher Education* (Princeton, N.J.: Princeton University Press, 2003).

Not only do research-intensive medical schools borrow heavily against anticipated income streams from academic-industrial partnerships, they also leverage their anticipated revenues from patient care. According to a 2004 survey by the American Association of Medical Colleges, "hard" revenues from tuition and endowment make up less than 10 percent of the average medical school's budget. In 1983, in comparison, "hard" revenues typically supported 60 to 70 percent of their budgets. Increasingly, medical schools are quietly readjusting their missions in favor of expansions into high-revenue patient care activities and reduction of low-margin activities, such as diabetes management clinics (see Ian Urbina, "In the Treatment of Diabetes, Success Often Does Not Pay," *The New York Times*, January 11, 2006). Several universities are hiring consultants who specialize in remaking academic tenure so as to reward faculty members participating in academic-industrial partnerships or emphasizing high-margin procedures and to penalize those who do not.

1: Trials of the Body

16   *Should you happen to look at Internet websites:* Specific cancers tend to have one or more websites, and Google and Yahoo are efficient at finding them. Some of them are patient-organized support and information groups. Pharmaceutical companies with new cancer drugs, such as Genentech, also maintain cancer treatment websites. Although many find them useful, cor-

porate websites tend to emphasize positive accounts of their new treatments. For general information on cancer, the following websites provide reams of useful information:

American Cancer Society: www.cancer.org

National Cancer Institute: www.cancer.gov

CATCHUM Project (Cancer Teaching and Curriculum Enhancement in Undergraduate Medicine): www.acor.org

Centers for Disease Control and Prevention—Cancer Information: www.cdc.gov/health/cancer.htm

24   *Did they find it significant, I continued:* The canons of Lateran Council IV (1215) are quoted in Dyan Elliott, *Proving Woman: Female Spirituality and Inquisitional Culture in the Later Middle Ages* (Princeton, N.J.: Princeton University Press, 2004).

3: Illusions of Control

54   *When a middle-aged man clutches his chest: Ambulance Doctor,* a film produced by Roosevelt Hospital, New York City, 1950. In film archive of History of Medicine Division, National Library of Medicine, Bethesda, Md.

57   *In comparison with any populous society:* For a contemporary Buddhist's exposition of "having" and "being," see Stephen Batchelor, *Alone with Others* (New York: Grove Press, 1983). In his *The Courage to Be* (London: Fontana, 1962), Paul Tillich, the Christian existentialist, provides a complementary view. On human experience, Michel de Montaigne's *Essays* has been a touchstone for me.

64   *At first glance, determining "medical futility," as the circumstance has become known:* The phrase *medical futility* dates from 1987. For a review article, see Paul R. Helft, Mark Siegler, and John Lantos, "The Rise and Fall of the Futility Movement," *New England Journal of Medicine* 343 (July 27, 2000):293–96.

69   *Ellen experienced ICU psychosis or delirium:* ICU psychosis is thought to be an acute organic disease of the brain associated with confinement in an ICU or similar setting. Affected patients become temporarily psychotic—that is, they experience intense anxiety and visual and auditory hallucinations.

71   *What Bentham particularly liked about his "Panopticon":* I find the full title of Bentham's work telling: *Panopticon: Or The Inspection-House: Containing the Idea of a New Principle of Construction Applicable to Any Sort of Establishment, in*

Which Persons of Any Description Are to be Kept Under Inspection; And in Particular to Penitentiary-Houses, Prisons, Houses of Industry, Work-Houses, Poor-Houses, Lazarettos, Manufactories, Hospitals, Mad-Houses, and Schools with a Plan of Management Adapted to the Principle: In a Series of Letters, Written in the Year 1787, From Crecheff in White Russia to a Friend in England by Jeremy Bentham, of Lincoln's Inn, Esquire. See Jeremy Bentham, *The Panopticon Writings,* ed. Miran Bozovic (London: Verso, 1995).

73   *In 1978 she founded a nonprofit organization, Planetree:* The Planetree website is www.Planetree.org.

4: Elective Choices

79   *During the 1980s, a Swiss demographer, Arthur Imhof:* For an English version of Imhof's work, see Arthur E. Imhof, "The Implications of Increased Life Expectancy for Family and Social Life," trans. Elizabeth Rusden, in Andrew Wear, ed., *Medicine in Society: Historical Essays* (New York: Cambridge University Press, 1992), pp. 347–74.

86   *Known as the Dartmouth Atlas of Health Care, these regularly updated maps:* On "more is not better," see John E. Wennberg, "Variation in Use of Medicare Services among Regions and Selected Academic Medical Centers: Is More Better?," the 2005 Duncan Clark Lecture of the New York Academy of Medicine, available on the Dartmouth Atlas website, www.dartmouthatlas.org. The Dartmouth Atlas project has received long-term funding from the Robert Wood Johnson Foundation.

89   *According to Dartmouth Atlas data, what determines:* On relationships between concentration of specialists and outcomes, see Katherine Baicker and Amitabh Chandra, "Medicare Spending, the Physician Workforce, and Beneficiaries' Quality of Care," *Health Affairs,* April 7, 2004, pp. 184–97.

94   *When it comes to the end of life—someone's last six months—the regional variation:* On variations in hospital care at the end of life, see *Health Affairs* webcast of October 7, 2005, available on the Dartmouth Atlas website.

95   *Elliott Fisher's group at Dartmouth and other studies:* Elliott Fisher, M.D., as quoted in *Dartmouth Medicine,* summer 2005, p. 29.

5: Reflections on the Plight of Sick Children

111   *In the mid-1970s a sociology graduate student:* Myra Bluebond Langer published her study as *Private Worlds of Dying Children* (Princeton, N.J.: Princeton University Press, 1980).

113   *Indeed, in the United States from the late 1800s:* On the history of child labor in the United States, see V. A. Zelzer, *Pricing the Priceless Child* (New York:

Basic Books, 1985). For a glimpse of mid-Victorian and Progressive-era medical attitudes to children, see Robert L. Martensen, "The Emergence of the Science of Childhood," *Journal of the American Medical Association* 275, no. 8 (1996):649.

117 *Perceptions, if not biomedical reality, took a turn:* The photo image on the cover of the current (fourth) edition of *A Child Is Born* (New York: Delacorte, 2003) is of a fetus at twenty-four weeks that appears to be in its own world, as neither its containing womb nor its mother is shown. The photograph opposite the title page, also intrauterine, is of a fetus at forty-six days.

120 *Echoing what Fost had found:* See Raymond S. Duff and A.G.M. Campbell, "Moral and Ethical Dilemmas in the Special-Care Nursery," *New England Journal of Medicine* 289 (October 25, 1973):890–94. For background on the "Baby Doe" regulations, see President's Commission for the Study of Ethical Problems in Medicine and Biomedical and Behavioral Research, *Deciding to Forego Life-Sustaining Treatment: Ethical, Medical, and Legal Issues in Treatment Decisions* (Washington, D.C.: U.S. Government Printing Office, 1983). The regulations themselves were included in the Child Abuse Amendments of 1984, 42 U.S.C.A. § 5102.

121 *Promoted enthusiastically by President Reagan:* The website for the President's Council on Bioethics, which is www.bioethics.gov, offers a vigorous discussion on bioethics and children by Norman Fost and others in the transcript for December 8, 2005, "Session 1: Bioethics and American Children."

6: If This Is a Person

132 *Dr. Fred Plum, the coauthor of a short text:* Plum's original description is in B. Jennett and F. Plum, "Persistent Vegetative State after Brain Damage: A Syndrome in Search of a Name," *Lancet* 1 (1972):734–37.

141 *At the conference he noted the following:* Robert Desjarlais's remarks were published in his commentary "On the Vagaries of Bodies," in *Culture, Medicine and Psychiatry* 19, no. 2 (1995):207–15. My presentation was published in the same issue as "Alienation and the Production of Strangers: Western Medical Epistemology and the Architectonics of the Body" (141–82). Desjarlais published his Nepalese study as *Body and Emotion: The Aesthetics of Illness and Healing in the Nepalese Himalayas* (Philadelphia: University of Pennsylvania Press, 1992). I published a history of Western attitudes toward the brain and personhood as *The Brain Takes Shape: An Early History* (New York: Oxford University Press, 2004).

144 *A few years later, in 1977, a prominent American:* John Knowles, "The Responsibility of the Individual," *Daedalus* 106 (winter 1977):57–80.

146   *A British anesthesiologist faced the issue head-on:* The anesthesiologist's observation is in Lesley Sharp's *Strange Harvest: Organ Transplants, Denatured Bodies and the Transformed Self* (Berkeley: University of California Press, 2006). Ian Hacking reviews the general subject and Sharp's book in his "Whose Body Is It?," *London Review of Books*, December 14, 2006, pp. 8–10.

147   *As a society we need to engage in reasonable discussions:* For a cognitive psychologist's assessment of current scientific understanding of consciousness, see Steven Pinker, "The Mystery of Consciousness," in *Time* magazine's "Mind and Body Special Issue" of January 29, 2007.

7: Life in the Narrows

159   *In the old days, before Mass Mental shut down:* For a history of community health centers, see Jessamy Taylor, "The Fundamentals of Community Health Centers," National Health Policy Forum Background Paper, August 31, 2004 (available online at www.nhpf.org). For a history of federal mental health policy, see Gerald N. Grob and Howard H. Goldman, *The Dilemma of Federal Mental Health Policy: Radical Reform or Incremental Change?* (New Brunswick, N.J.: Rutgers University Press, 2007).

163   *These structures constitute the endangered ecology of community health:* For an overview of how narrow considerations of financial interest have led medical centers to downplay disease management clinics in favor of expanding high-margin specialist offerings, see the four-part series "The Business of Care," in *The New York Times*, January 2006.

164   *As of 2005, the entire federal budget request:* For Bush administration's 2005 budget request of $1.79 billion for support of community health centers, see Taylor, "The Fundamentals of Community Health Centers."

8: As Night Draws Nigh

190   *In short, "justification by double effect . . . may function as a 'fig leaf' for euthanasia":* The fig leaf characterization is from Truog, Berde, Mitchell, and Grier, "Barbiturates in the Care of the Terminally Ill," *New England Journal of Medicine* 327 (1992):1678–80.

190   *If you are approaching death in New York:* For an extensive discussion of New York State laws and why some patients and physicians object to them, see "*Vacco* v. *Quill* Brief," available online at www.compassionindying.org. Quill's statement is from p. 11. Subsequently, the U.S. Supreme Court upheld the New York law that Quill et al. were appealing. A brief online account of the Court's position by Joan Biskupic, "Unanimous Decision Points to Tradition

of Valuing Life" (June 27, 1997), at www.washingtonpost.com. See also T. E. Quill, R. Dresser, and D. W. Brock, "The Rule of Double Effect—A Critique of Its Role in End-of-Life Decision Making," *New England Journal of Medicine* 337 (December 11, 1997):1768–71.

193 *The late Pope John Paul II could not have been clearer:* John Paul's remarks are from his "Address of John Paul II to the Participants in the International Congress on Life-Sustaining Treatments and Vegetative State: Scientific Advances and Ethical Dilemmas," March 20, 2004, available online at www.vatican.va.

Acknowledgments

During my time in college in New England, I wrote and published several short stories, took a broad array of courses, and majored in design. I thought about going into medicine, but I did not want to experience college as a premed. Two years out of college and broke in Albuquerque, I began working as a hospital janitor. As I cleaned up ORs and patients' rooms, the notion of being a doctor returned and grew. Fortunately, the University of New Mexico then had a nondegree path that allowed one to take a full load of science courses for two hundred dollars a year. I signed up, enjoyed the experience, and a year later found myself accepted as a "nontraditional" medical student at Dartmouth. In those days I imagined I would go into family practice in Vermont and write stories on the side. Like others with medical and literary inclinations, my models were William Carlos Williams and Anton Chekhov. Instead of staying in New England, however, I went to San Francisco for residency, stayed for twenty years in its midst, and barely wrote a fictive word.

Around the time of my fortieth birthday, I decided I would go back into the humanities, this time into history. The University of California at San Francisco and Berkeley had a small but superb program in the history of medicine and science, and I found I could combine part-time ER work with full-time graduate school. Upon graduation in 1993, when academic jobs were scarce, I felt lucky to be offered a position in Boston that combined history with medical practice.

Since graduate school, I have written numerous historical articles and one book—*The Brain Takes Shape: An Early History*—intended primarily for physicians, scientists, and professional historians. Even so, my muse as a writer has always been what Virginia Woolf termed "the common reader." Two people have given me an opportunity to engage that muse with this book. I met Susan Arellano, my agent, through the Internet. Her business partner at the time, Susan Rabiner, had cowritten with Albert Fortunato, her husband, an immensely useful book on writing nonfiction, *Thinking Like Your Editor.* When I e-mailed the Rabiner agency with a book idea after reading her writing guide, Susan Arellano e-mailed back. Since then, Susan A., who is now with InkWell Management, has been unflagging in her patience and astute in her comments. I should add that we worked on proposals for more than a year before she suggested that one was ready for submission. We do our business on a handshake. I hope all writers are as fortunate.

Eric Chinski, my editor at Farrar, Straus and Giroux, has been a dream to work with. Even when he has been overwhelmed with other matters, Eric has made the time for open-ended conversations about this book and questions it raises. He edits like the deftest of surgeons, careful to tease out lesions that need excision without damaging surrounding tissues or causing an author much loss of blood.

When I started writing this book in July 2005, I thought my life was settled. I had completed renovation of my home, a boathouse on Lake Ponchartrain in New Orleans; my sons and I had just spent glorious weeks in Barcelona and London; and I had a wonderful circle of local friends. Then Katrina blew in. When I was able to return to New Orleans in November, I found my home and community destroyed. During the interim, I stayed in New York City, where Jerry Barondess and his colleagues at the New York Academy of Medicine went out of their way to make me feel welcome with an office and congenial company. New York friends, including Bill Helfand, Roger Kent, and Craig Wern, loaned me their guest rooms and apartments and did much to ease my despair. I owe them and others deep thanks.

Among physicians and ethicists, Adam Asch, George Ho, Loretta Kopelman, Janet Malek, and Mitt Seiler have provided valuable comments and corrections. John Barry, Dawn Dedeaux, and Anne Sullivan of New Orleans have given sound advice, as have Pia Pera in Italy, Bill and Helen Bynum in England, and Noga Arikha and Marcello Simonetti in New York. Noga's generous and expert line edit of a draft has improved the final text immensely. Friends Matt McGarvey, Iva Gourguieva, Maggie Kent, and Huston Paschal read early versions and asked useful questions. Andy Baxter, who lost his wife, Carley Cunniff, to cancer in 2005, has made me feel this book serves a real purpose. My children—Bayard, Charlie, and Max—have provided encouragement from beginning to end.

Index

survival with, 12–13, 15, 17, 19, 20, 23; radiation treatment of, 10, 11, 12, 19, 20; research and advances in, 13, 18–20; surgical treatment of, 8–11, 19–20, 92; symptoms of, 5–7
breasts: examination of, 5–7, 9; infection of, 6, 7
breathing: arrest of, 67, 135, 139, 148, 183, 185; difficulties with, ix, xi, 67, 68, 78, 81, 88, 90, 175, 177, 178, 180, 182, 184, 187; medical management of, *see* breathing tubes; oxygen, supplemental; ventilators
breathing tubes, 67, 68, 69, 135, 185; *see also* ventilators
bronchitis, 61, 159, 176
Brownback, Sam, 27
Buddhism, 131, 140–41
Bush, George W., 165

California, University of: at Los Angeles (UCLA), 95; at San Francisco (UCSF), 95
Campion, Rosamund, 19–20
cancer, ix, 90, 92, 114; American vs. European treatments for, 26; childhood, 18, 104–108; death from, 10, 12, 19, 22–23, 27, 48, 109, 148; metastatic, 3–4, 5–13, 18–23, 31, 35, 38, 45, 46, 47, 49–50, 105, 174; predictable downward course of, 48, 51, 173, 174; remission of, 11, 17, 23, 115; solid, 12, 18, 23, 35, 46, 50, 84, 104–105; Stage IV, 12, 38, 45, 94, 96, 173–74; surgery for,

8–9, 19–20, 36, 37, 38, 40, 49, 84, 105, 106; theories about, 19; *see also* tumors; *specific cancers*
cancer centers, 16, 20
cancer phobias, 35
cancer specialists, 7, 8, 10, 20, 36, 39–40, 44, 104–105, 110
cancer teams, 10, 27, 105
carbohydrates, 165
carbon dioxide, 125–26
cardiac bypass pumps, 82, 84, 85, 88
cardiac defibrillators, 79
cardiac surgery, 36, 81–85, 87
cardiology, 81–85, 89, 101
cardiovascular disease, *see* heart disease
CARE, 7
catheters, 62, 67, 70–71, 126, 186
Catholic Church, *see* Roman Catholic Church
CAT scans, 12, 15, 35, 40, 131, 134
chaplains, 68–69
chemotherapy, 36, 49–50; aggressive, 12, 18, 19–21; experimental, 10, 12–17, 22–23, 27–28; multiple rounds of, 9, 10, 99, 105; overall survival and, 12–13, 15, 17; palliative, 50; quality of life and, 13; side effects and toxicity of, 12, 13, 14–15, 18, 20, 28, 115–16
chest: emergency opening of, 40, 64; pain in, 92, 99, 160–61; tubes in, 37–38, 56
Chicago White Sox, 93
Child Abuse Prevention and Treatment Act of 1984, 121
children: death as seen by, 111; death of, 109, 111, 112, 115–16, 119, 121; dignity and personhood of,

137–38, 147; transplantation of, 122, 126–27, 136–38, 140, 147

organ transplant coordinators, 126–27, 135, 136–37, 147

orthopedists, 89–90, 125

Our Bodies, Ourselves, 118

Oxfam, 7

Oxford English Dictionary, 3

oxygen: blood, 125–26, 175, 177, 178, 182; prompt administration of, 54, 55, 166; supplemental, 51, 82, 175, 177, 178, 180, 183

pain: cancer, 50–51; surgical, 38, 40

pain medicine, 13, 25–26, 38, 50, 180

palliative care, 13, 25–26, 28, 36, 44, 51, 94, 105, 109, 174; chemotherapy in, 50; surgical, 36, 45–46; *see also* hospice care

panic, 68

Panopticon, 71–72, 74

paralysis, 128, 129–30

paramedics, 77, 177, 185

patients, 53–56; advanced directives of, 41, 123, 175, 179–80, 185, 186–87, 192; autonomy of, 55–56, 66, 69–70; conservative treatments preferred by, 91–92; as consumers, 55–56, 58; hospital discharge initiated by, 69–70; medical advocacy for, 108–109, 119–23; natural healing tendency of, 59, 70; prisoners compared to, 71–72; proactive participation of, 56; relapses of, 69; relationships of physicians and, 3, 37, 66, 90–91, 104–106; sense of entitlement in,

58; sources of medical information available to, ix, 16, 20, 33, 56, 73–74, 86, 90, 92; surrogates of, 65

peau d'orange, see breast cancer, inflammatory

pediatric care, 104, 114–16, 119–23, 135, 151

persistent vegetative state (PVS), 126–27, 135, 145–47, 193; coma vs., 132; conditions leading to, 139–40; minimal consciousness and, 140, 146, 147; prolonged medical attention in, 142–43

personhood, xii, 91, 144; body and, 140–41; of children, 102–104, 120; definitions of, xii, 140–43, 146, 155–56; diminishment of, 57, 70; recovery of, 72–73, 75; soul and, 140–41

PET scans, 131

pharmaceutical companies, 16–17, 27; representatives of, 159

physical examinations, 5–7, 9, 30–31

physicians: advertising by, 56; as advocates for patient welfare, 108–11, 119–23, 136–37; delivery of diagnosis to patients by, 6–7, 31–32; disagreement among, 62–63, 65; disclosure obligations of, 13, 83–85; emergency, x, 4–6, 9, 20–23, 31, 33, 34, 46, 82, 90, 139, 158–62; emotional involvement of, 6, 145; in group practice, 101; lawsuits against, 82–85, 110–11; legal power of, 70, 106–107; medieval, 24; patients' demands as seen by, 110–11; patients' mental competence determined by, 69, 70;